THE CLINICAL APPLICATION OF MMPI SPECIAL SCALES

Second Edition

THE CLINICAL APPLICATION OF MMPI SPECIAL SCALES

Second Edition

Eugene E. Levitt, Ph. D.

Indiana University School of Medicine

Edward E. Gotts, Ph. D.

Madison (Indiana) State Hospital

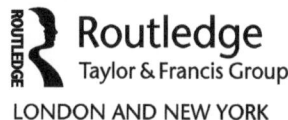

Routledge
Taylor & Francis Group

LONDON AND NEW YORK

First published 1995 by Lawrence Erlbaum Associates, Inc.

Published 2020 by Routledge
2 Park Square, Milton Park, Abingdon, Oxon OX14 4RN
605 Third Avenue, New York, NY 10017

First issued in paperback 2021

Routledge is an imprint of the Taylor & Francis Group, an informa business

Library of Congress Cataloging-in-Publication Data

Levitt, Eugene E.
    The clinical application of MMPI special scales / Eugene E.
Levitt, Edward E. Gotts. — 2nd ed.
        p.   cm.
    Includes bibliographical references and indexes.
    ISBN 0–8058–1770–0 (hard : alk. paper)
    1. Minnesota Multiphasic Personality Inventory.   2. Mental
illness—Diagnosis.   3. Adjustment (Psychology)—Testing.
    I. Gotts, Edward Earl.   II. Title.
    [DNLM: 1. MMPI.   2. Personality Assessment.   3. Mental Disorders-
-diagnosis.   WM 145 L666c   1995]
    RC473.M5L48   1995
    616.89′075—dc20
    DNLM/DLC
    for Library of Congress   94–39481
                                                                  CIP

ISBN 13: 978-1-138-98891-0 (pbk)
ISBN 13: 978-0-8058-1770-6 (hbk)
ISBN 13: 978-1-315-82742-1 (ebk)

DOI: 10.4324/9781315827421

CONTENTS

PREFACE
TO THE SECOND EDITION

Like all revisions that strive to be worthy, this second edition examines and assesses the relevant literature that has appeared since the publication of the first edition. Meaningful recent investigations have been included in the text, in some instances supplanting older ones.

This second edition, however, is more than simply an update. It has three entirely new features. One of these is the innovative, so-called Human Computer Program, a library of diagnostic statements based on MMPI special scales and individual items that are cast in a form suitable for writing reports or for creating a computer narrative program. Another innovation is the first comprehensive attempt to diagnose personality disorders from special scales and items. The publication of MMPI–2 in the interim between editions is recognized in several ways. The MMPI–2 content scales, the only special scales created from the MMPI–2 pool to date, are discussed in the context of the original MMPI content scales. The impact of MMPI–2 on the main cohort of special scales is also discussed with a demonstration of their continued usefulness within MMPI–2 records.

The authors wish to express their gratitude to Lisa Partlow for her important role in the preparation of the manuscript of this monograph.

We have prepared profile forms that will facilitate use of the interpretive system in the Human Computer Program, Appendix V in this book. For further information and sample profile forms, write to: Edward E. Gotts, Ph.D., 711 Green Road, Madison, IN 47250.

Edward E. Gotts
Eugene E. Levitt

SPECIAL SCALES KEY

Harris & Lingoes Scales

2SD = Subjective Depression
2PR = PsychomotorRetardation
2PM = PhysicalMalfunctioning
2MD = Mental Dullness
2B = Brooding
3DSA = Denial of Social Anxiety
3NA = Need for Affection
3LM = Lassitude and Malaise
3SC = Somatic Complaints
3IA = Inhibition of Aggression
4FD = Familial Discord
4AC = Authority Conflict
4SI = Social Imperturbability
4SOA = Social Alienation
4SEA = Self-Alienation
6PI = Persecutory Ideas
6P = Poignancy
6N = Naivete
8SOA = Social Alienation
8EA = Emotional Alienation
8COG = Lack of Ego Mastery, Cognitive

8CON = Lack of Ego Mastery, Conative
8BSE = Bizarre Sensory Experiences
8DIC = Lack of Ego Mastery, Defect of Inhibition and Control
9AMO = Amorality
9PMA = Psychomotor Acceleration
9EI = Ego Inflation
9IMP = Imperturbability

Wiggins Scales

AUT = Authority Conflict
DEP = Depression
FAM = Family Problems
FEM = Feminine Interests
HEA = Poor Health
HYP = Hypomania
HOS = Manifest Hostility
MOR = Poor Morale
ORG = Organic Symptoms
PHO = Phobias
PSY = Psychoticism
REL = Religious Fundamentalism
SOC = Social Maladjustment

Tryon, Stein, & Chu Scales

TSC/A = Autism
TSC/B = Body Symptoms
TSC/D = Depression
TSC/I = Social Introversion
TSC/R = Resentment
TSC/S = Suspicion
TSC/T = Tension

Indiana Scales

I-De = Dependency
I-Do = Dominance
I-DS = Dissociative Symptoms
I-OC = Obsessive-Compulsiveness
I-RD = Severe Reality Distortions
I-SC = Self-Concept
I-SP = Sex Problems

Other Scales

AMac = MacAndrew Alcoholism Scale
Astvn = Assertiveness
CLS = Carelessness
Cn = Control
D-S = Depression, Subtle
E/Cy = Cynicism
Ho = Hostility
ME = Mean Evaluation on eight clinical scales
OH = Overcontrolled Hostility
S+ = Extreme Suspiciousness
TR = Test-Retest
WA = Work Attitude
5C = Conventionality
Pe = Pedophilia

CHAPTER 1
INTRODUCTION

Many verbal inventories for the measurement of psychopathology and personality have been developed over the past 40 years. Some attained modest prominence at least for a time; others were neglected from the beginning and little is known about their attributes and capacities. Only a handful have survived perennially. The outstanding example is the Minnesota Multiphasic Personality Inventory (MMPI). The original MMPI was created 50 years ago but remains the most popular formal assessment tool in psychology and education. It has the deepest potential for evaluating human personality, for measuring change in personal and emotional status, for increasing the accuracy of diagnosis, and for giving useful information regarding treatment plans and prognosis. Thousands of publications, perennial workshops, and computerized interpretive programs testify to the popularity of the MMPI. An estimated 15 million MMPIs are administered in the United States alone each year.

Despite its longevity, the MMPI has a number of methodological defects that have been summarized by Faschingbauer (1979) and Levitt and Duckworth (1984). Wiener and Harmon (1946) observed early that there are two types of statements in the MMPI clinical scales; obvious and subtle. An obvious item is one for which the psychopathological or diagnostic response is clear as, for example, responding "true" to the statement "Life is a strain for me much of the time." A subtle item is one for which there is no response that is keyed for psychopathology as, for example, "I like *Alice in Wonderland* by Lewis Carroll."

Every relevant investigation has shown that the correlations between the obvious and subtle subsections of the clinical scales range from zero to low negative, a certain mathematical argument for dimensional independence. Summing these unrelated subsets into a single score can only be a "cancellation approach" to scale scores (Norman, 1972; Faschingbauer, 1979).

The obvious–subtle differential is not the only criticism that has been leveled at MMPI clinical scales. Faschingbauer (1979) described them as "heterogeneous, redundant, and overlapping . . . over 100 items are not even scored. How much potentially useful information never enters the code type as a result is still unknown" (p. 374). Faschingbauer is in essential agreement with Norman (1972) who pointed out that the clinical scales are not only "inefficient, redundant, and largely irrelevant for their present purposes" (p. 64) but also the MMPI methods of "combining scale scores and for profile interpretation are unconscionably cumbersome and obtuse" (p. 64). Norman summed up by noting that "it is abundantly clear that they are about as inappropriate and maladapted a set as one could imagine for their current uses in profile analysis, and interpretation and typal class definition" (p. 64). Archer and Krishnamurthy (1993b) theorize that the general absence of correlation between the MMPI and the Rorschach "could be the result of the multidimensional nature of most of the basic MMPI clinical scales" (p. 286).

Wiggins (1966), commenting on the heterogeneity of the clinical scales, remarked that "the hodgepodge of content which contributes to a high score on a given clinical scale is not suggestive of any consistent personality trait or structure" (p. 31). Indeed, the libraries of interpretive statements that have been proposed for high scores on clinical scales are at best unenlightening and at worst, confusing. For example, Graham (1987) listed 44 interpretive statements that can accompany a high score on Scale 4 plus 16 statements that follow from low scores. A high score on Scale 9 yields 42 interpretive statements, a low score, 14 more. Clopton (1979a) pointed out the obvious: Respondents endorsing very different subsets of items can obtain the same raw score on any scale.

Thus, to select the appropriate interpretative statements from among Graham's lists requires that the clinician examine the protocol's individual item responses. It is unsafe to make interpretations based solely on the clinical scale score.

To exemplify this phenomenon, Wiggins (1966) created profiles for two hypothetical patients whose clinical scale profiles (see Fig. 1.1) were identical but whose scores on Wiggins' content scales varied markedly as indicated in Table 1.1.

Obviously, the interpretations of the two identical clinical profiles using high point codes or any other method of analysis would also be identical. Wiggins discussed the differences in interpretation of the two records according to Table 1.1.

Patient A has admitted to a larger number of symptoms thought to be indicative of organic pathology. Additionally, he admits having family problems and a number of psychotic symptoms of a primarily paranoid nature. He is greatly concerned

TABLE 1.1
Raw Scores on Wiggins Scales for Two Hypothetical Patients
with Identical Clinical Scale Profiles

Content scale	Patient A	Patient B	Difference
ORG	28	5	+23
PSY	8	21	−13
HEA	7	20	−13
FEM	6	17	−11
FAM	11	6	+5
DEP	15	19	−4
HYP	8	12	−4
PHO	13	9	+4
SOC	10	13	−3
HOS	9	12	−3
AUT	13	11	+2
REL	7	9	−2
MOR	12	11	+1

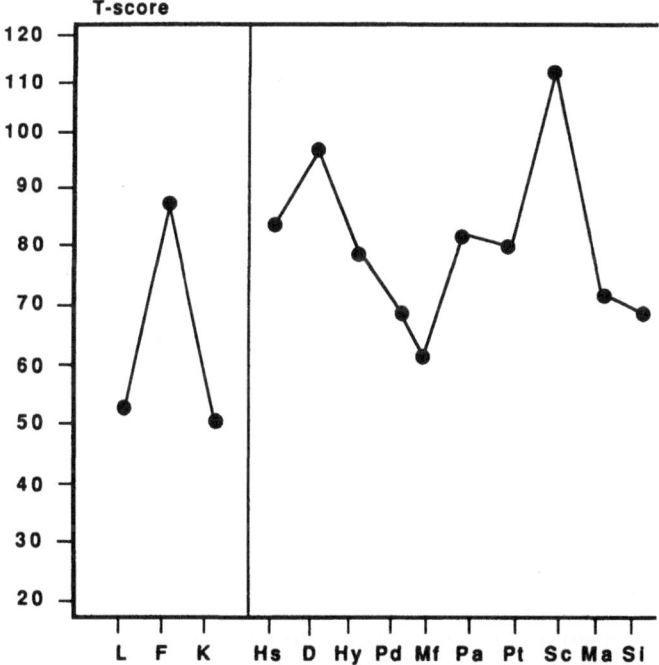

FIG. 1.1. Clinical profile of Wiggins' hypothetical patients.

3

about his health and admits to liking an unusual number of feminine pursuits. By comparison with Patient A, Patient B is generally more deviant with respect to content categories reflecting poor morale, mood instability, social maladjustment and hostility.

The configuration of content scale scores of Patient B readily confirms the impression of psychopathology gained from an inspection of the clinical profile in Figure 1.1. This could be the profile of a paranoid schizophrenic with an underlying homosexual component and a body concern that is delusional in nature. Poor morale, social maladjustment, and hostility are, of course, compatible with this picture.

Although Patient A's raw content scale scores are sufficiently deviant to be considered those of a hospitalized patient, they are in sharp contrast to those of Patient B. By comparison, Patient A is almost exclusively concerned with organic symptoms and, to a lesser extent, family problems. Evidence of delusional thinking, health concern, feminine interests, and general maladjustment is comparatively weak for Patient A. The clinical scale profile in Figure 1.1 may now be viewed in a quite different light. (Wiggins, 1966, p. 30)

The MMPI clinical scales are not without their defenders. The thrust of the defense is that the clinical scales were intended to measure psychopathology, not personality traits and it is unfair to criticize the MMPI for being unable to do what it has never been intended to do (Dahlstrom, 1969; Butcher & Tellegen, 1978).

Thus, Dahlstrom (1969) pointed out that internal item consistency and homogeneity are not relevant to the task of the MMPI. The important criterion, according to Dahlstrom, is not whether an item correlates with other items but whether it improves clinical prediction about patient groups (i.e., external rather than internal validity).

Dahlstrom added that the obvious and subtle dimensions of clinical scales are relatively uncorrelated among normal persons but have much higher correlations for appropriate psychiatric patient reference groups.

As we see here, the issue of the intent of the MMPI is actually irrelevant but for purposes of completeness of the argument, it might be noted that the original purpose of the MMPI may not be as clearcut as Dahlstrom (1969) and Butcher and Tellegen (1978) suggest. Consider the following quotations from the original MMPI *Manual* (Hathaway & McKinley, 1951):

The Minnesota Multiphasic Personality Inventory is a psychometric instrument designed ultimately to provide, in a single test, scores on all the more important phases of personality. The point of view determining the importance of a trait in this case is that of the clinical or personnel worker who wished to assay those traits that are commonly characteristic of disabling psychological abnormality . . . personality characteristics may be assessed on the basis of scores on nine clinical scales originally developed for use with the Inventory . . . although the scales are named according to the abnormal manifestation of the symptomatic complex, they have all been shown to have meaning within the normal range . . . as for validity, a high score on a scale has been found to predict positively the corresponding final clinical diagnosis or estimate in more than 60 percent of new psychiatric admissions. (pp. 5–6)

Thus, it appears on the one hand, the constructors of the MMPI are saying that the instrument is intended for differential diagnosis among psychiatric patients and on the other, that scale scores also measure personality characteristics of normal persons.

The most recent edition of the original MMPI *Manual* (Hathaway & McKinley, 1983) had less to say about the intent of the instrument, possibly with the thought that it is by now so well known that a statement of purpose is almost gratuitous. The *Manual*'s opening sentences state that the MMPI "is designed to provide an objective assessment of some of the major personality characteristics that affect personal and social adjustment. The point of view determining the importance of a trait in this case is that of the clinical or personnel worker who wishes to assay those traits that are commonly characteristic of disabling psychological abnormality" (p. 1). No further comment is made beyond this succinct bit of weaseling which still leaves unsettled the not too important issue of whether Hathaway and McKinley intended to create a personality inventory or a diagnostic instrument.

Despite the item amendments that constitute the revised version of the MMPI, MMPI-2, the original clinical scales survived almost intact (Butcher, Dahlstrom, Graham, Tellegen & Kaemmer, 1989). This "continuity between the original MMPI and its revision" was the intent of the revision committee (Graham, 1990, p. 9). An obvious inference is that most of the criticisms of the original MMPI clinical scales apply as well to the clinical scales of MMPI-2. (For a general critique of MMPI-2, see Duckworth & Levitt, 1994).

Fortunately, the MMPI clinical scales are not the only available groupings of MMPI items. Over the years, psychologists working with the original MMPI devised a substantial number of scales composed of MMPI items. Four methods for developing new measures have been employed:

1. Cluster and factor analyses of the total MMPI pool (e.g., Eichman, 1961, 1962).

2. Ratios of various clinical scales like the Index of Psychopathology (Sines & Silver, 1963) and the Anxiety Index and Internalization Ratio (Welsh, 1952).

3. Content scales based on selection of items by clinical judgment like the Manifest Anxiety Scale (Taylor, 1953).

4. Empirical selection of items usually based on a comparison of contrasting groups. This procedure has furnished by far the bulk of all the special scales that have been developed from the MMPI pool over the years.

The first edition of Volume I of the MMPI *Handbook* (Dahlstrom & Welsh, 1960) listed 213 special scales and ratios that had been constructed from the MMPI pool. The second edition of this volume (Dahlstrom, Welsh, & Dahlstrom, 1975) contained 455 special scales and ratios. A few years later, Butcher and Tellegen (1978) suggested that there were more special scales than items!

Neglect of the Special Scales

Unfortunately, there is only scanty information on the large majority of special scales. Megargee and Mendelsohn (1962) point out that:

> The clinical researcher who wishes to measure some aspect of personality by using one of these scales often has little information about their real meaning or usefulness. A search of the literature generally reveals little data on which to base a decision for the amount of cross-validation is too often nonexistent or inadequate. Frequently the only information available is that which Dahlstrom and Welsh (1960) have gleaned from unpublished sources, or the title which the scalemaker has given to his instrument. The question naturally arises as to how valid these scales are and whether their publication represents progress or merely additional noise in the field. (pp. 431–432)

The development of MMPI special scales often demonstrates "a lack of conceptual clarity," according to Clopton (1979a, p. 365). He added that this criticism "applies to the naming of newly developed scales, the selection of criterion and comparison groups, and the intended use of the new scale" (p. 365). Butcher and Tellegen (1978) note further that:

> Many scales have been constructed by contrasting different "samples of convenience" (often of heterogeneous makeup or with important characteristics unknown). Often these scales are not cross-validated and more often than not their psychometric properties and inter-relations with other scales are not reported. Many new scales, since they are, after all, derived from the same item pool, prove to be largely redundant alternative versions of existing scales, although sometimes of poorer quality. (p. 622)

Cross-validation or replication is a crucial step in test construction because of the ever-present problem of sampling error and the inevitable possibility of sample bias. If we draw two samples from the same population, we should not expect on purely logical grounds, that *any* MMPI items would significantly differentiate the samples. But it will almost always occur that *some* items, perhaps as many as 5% of them, will indeed be differentially responded to by the two samples. We recognize this as a chance occurrence, a function of uncontrolled variables. If we then select a second pair of samples from the same population, we should again expect that about 5% of the items will significantly differentiate the two samples but not by any means the same ones as in the first pair of samples.

In the contrasting groups methods of test construction, the two samples are defined as representing different populations according to some variable or variables: sex, age, race, diagnosis, and so on. But they nonetheless represent the same population with respect to the dependent variable that defines the desired measuring instrument (i.e., Sickly Shyness or Robust Extraversion or High Back Pain). Nevertheless, there should be differentiating MMPI items as a sheer function of chance. To test the possibility that this outcome has undermined the test construction, a replication of the investigation is requisite—a cross-validation. If all or most of the original differentiating items are still differentiating in the replication, there is a good chance that a scale has been born. If not, the hypothesis of chance differentiation becomes paramount.

An excellent illustration of cross-validation technique and the need for it is the report by Lachar, Lewis, and Kupke (1979). They administered the MMPI to two small groups of epileptics who were classified as either temporal lobe or nontemporal lobe seizure types on the basis of seizure behavior and electroencephalographic findings. The groups were carefully matched for age, sex, race, education, intelligence, and general neuropsychological impairment. Analysis of the MMPI records revealed no differences between the two groups either on clinical scale scores or 2-point code types.

An item analysis identified 50 MMPI statements which distinguished the two groups. Scores on this set of items, which investigators less cautious than Lachar and his associates might have immediately called the Lobe Identification Scale for Epileptics (LISE), successfully distinguished all members of both groups. Lachar et al. now proceeded to select two new groups of temporal and nontemporal lobe epileptics that were descriptively similar to the original groups. Mean LISE scores obtained by these cross-validation samples were *not* statistically different. The authors conclude that the cross-validation failure "dramatically illustrates the scientific parsimony of successful cross-validation of any new classificatory scale before discussion of its function and item composition" (p. 187).

One can only suspect that a goodly number of the MMPI special scales listed in Dahlstrom et al. (1975) would fail the cross-validation test.

Both Megargee and Mendelsohn and Butcher and Tellegen caution that the title given to a special scale by its constructor may be misleading and should not be accepted uncritically. Again, unfortunately, the large majority of special scales have been inadequately researched to determine whether or not the construct title given to the scale by its constructor is applicable or misleading.

Discussion of the interpretation of special scales is uncommon. Graham (1987), Duckworth and Anderson (1986), and Greene (1991) are exceptions. Graham (1978) has also produced a scholarly review of the experimental findings with a number of the special scales and Clopton (1979a) has contributed a chapter on special scale construction. But there is too much space around these landmarks which doubtlessly explains the limited use of special scales by MMPI diagnosticians (Moreland & Dahlstrom, 1983).

The chronic neglect of the special scale is at least partly due to the conservatism of the major proponents of the MMPI. The usual MMPI workshop perennially presents endless research findings and clinical lore deriving from traditional high-point code typologies. Occasionally, there may be a brief mention of a special scale, usually one that appeared in the old *Basic Readings* compendium (Welsh & Dahlstrom, 1956). This neglect surely reached a nadir in an article on the future of the MMPI (Faschingbauer, 1979). In this 20-page prophecy, a single 15-word phrase is devoted to special scales!

Even some of those few who take note of the special scales seem to be oppressed by a peculiar ambivalence, perhaps tinged with guilt. Graham (1987), for example, felt obliged to warn his readers in three separate textual admonitions that the special scales "are viewed as supplementary to interpretation of the standard MMPI scales and should not be used instead of these standard scales" (p. 116). Duckworth and Anderson (1986), after a dozen years and three editions, have discovered only 14 of the myriad of special scales.

THE PURPOSE OF THIS BOOK

This book is intended to facilitate the clinical employment of MMPI special scales. They offer an abundance of information beyond that provided by the clinical scales and a precision that the clinical scales cannot match. No claim is made that the special scales have ironclad validity. Obviously, they do not, a testimonial to the absence of empirical research. But much the same can be said of high-point codes based on clinical scales. In fact, several large scale investigations strongly suggest that high-point code typologies are sorely lacking in utility (e.g., Palmer, 1970; Huff, 1965; Winters, Weintraub, & Neale, 1981). No solid experimental data supports the conventional high-point code typology. The widely used MMPI code type manuals (e.g., Gilberstadt & Duker, 1965; Marks & Seeman, 1963) are as clinically based as the interpretations offered in this book.

The few proponents of the use of special scales have been candid about the basis of their interpretive suggestions. Duckworth and Anderson (1986), in their chapter on interpretation of special scales, remark that because "little information about them has appeared in the research literature" their interpretations are "based primarily upon our own work in various counseling and clinical settings" (Duckworth & Anderson, 1986, p. 236). Graham (1987) and Greene (1980) in their MMPI volumes acknowledge "the author's own clinical experience," as Graham put it, as the fundament of special scale analysis.

The interpretations of special scales presented in this volume are also based primarily on clinical experience. What follows is a statement of the source and scope of that experience.

Clinical work with MMPI special scales began at the Indiana University Medical Center in 1969 when Dr. Robert Lushene, then at Florida State University, provided a computer program which scored approximately 115 special scales and ratios in addition to the conventional clinical scales. Over the next 15 years, this program and its several revisions scored somewhere near 70,000 MMPI records derived from more than 75 different populations on 155 scales and ratios. These included not only psychiatric and medical inpatients and outpatients but such diverse groups as applicants for law enforcement agencies, air traffic controllers, the clergy of several religious denominations, parents of children in child psychiatry clinics, applicants for surgical gender reassignment, candidates for various types of positions in industrial and organization settings, and research subjects. Some thousands of these individuals were in direct contact with clinical psychologists at the Indiana University Medical Center, either because the MMPI was part of a test battery, or because the testee was a patient of the psychologist or because the patient was presented as part of a diagnostic or treatment review conference. Some of the agencies outside of the Indiana University Medical Center that made use of the program provided feedback, either systematically or occasionally. All told, a large body of clinical data on a group of more than 150 MMPI special scales was accumulated[1]. Some of these measures were not found to be diagnostically applicable or to have limited utility (see Appendix VI). Those scales that survived the test of prolonged clinical employment form the fundament of this monograph. They are listed in Appendix I with their item content and sources.

The Indiana Sample

The two recent efforts to provide contemporary norms for the MMPI testify abundantly to its gerontological status. Data for the original normative sample of 724 subjects (Hathaway & McKinley, 1940) and the so-called refined sample of 541 subjects (Hathaway & Briggs, 1957) were collected before 1940. The first attempt at renorming was carried out by scientists at the Mayo Clinic in Minnesota (Colligan, Osborn, Swenson & Offord, 1983, 1989). No items were dropped or altered in this project. The most recent is the restandardization project that produced MMPI-2 (Butcher, et al., 1989.) In MMPI-2, 90 of the original items were discarded, 70 were altered and 107 new items were added (Butcher, et al., 1989; Levitt, 1990).

At about the same time, we collected a small sample of normal subjects to use in our computer program for scoring special scales. Our norms were already

[1]The psychologists who were primarily involved in the aggregation of this pool of information were Frank J. Connolly, Drs. Wm. George McAdoo, Nuran B. Miller and Charles W. Perkins, in addition to the senior author. Their unintentional but very necessary collaboration with the fundament of this book is gratefully acknowledged. Connolly also conceived of the acronym schema for the Harris and Lingoes (1968) and the Pepper and Strong (1958) subscales of the MMPI clinical scales. A major indebtedness to Dr. Robert Lushene for his seminal contribution is also acknowledged.

TABLE 1.2
A Comparison of Indiana Norms with MMPI-2[a] and Mayo Clinic[b] Norms
for MMPI Clinical and Validity Scales Using K-Uncorrected Raw Scores

	Males			Females		
Scale	Indiana	MMPI-2	Mayo	Indiana	MMPI-2	Mayo
1	5.7	4.9	5.5	7.2	5.9	5.9
2	18.7	18.3	18.9	20.4	20.1	21.2
3	19.2	20.9	20.0	21.2	22.1	21.4
4	17.1	16.6	15.2	16.6	16.2	14.4
5	24.6	26.0	24.4	37.1	35.9	38.3
6	9.9	10.1	9.5	10.1	10.2	9.8
7	12.7	11.2	11.3	13.2	12.7	12.1
8	12.9	11.2	10.4	13.0	11.2	9.6
9	18.9	16.9	15.8	17.7	16.1	14.1
0	26.1	25.9	27.8	29.8	28.0	30.1
L	4.0	3.5	3.8	3.8	3.6	4.1
F	6.5	4.5	4.5	5.3	3.7	3.6
K	14.7	15.3	14.2	12.8	15.0	14.8

[a]Data from Appendix B in Butcher, et al. (1989)
[b]Data from Appendix I in Colligan et al. (1983). The data are for the census-matched subsample.

in use at the time that the Colligan, et al. (1983) data were published. The sampling procedure we employed was modeled after Beck, Rabin, Thiesen, Molish, and Thetford (1950) who collected Rorschach normative data. An entrepreneur kindly makes available his entire staff for testing.[2] These include every literate employee ranging from unskilled laborers, through semi-skilled and skilled workers and office staff to executives. This provided a solid nucleus of 64 respondents. To this group were added 28 adult subjects from research projects and 18 soldiers[3]. Ten of these 110 subjects were discarded because the respondents omitted 30 items or more, or because TR + CLS was at least 7 (see Chapter 2). An effort had been made to have an equal sex ratio but the discarded records left 51 women and 49 men. The demographic characteristics of this sample are shown in Appendix II.

Most of the statistical statements concerning special scales that are made in this book, such as correlation coefficients, are based on the Indiana sample. Appendix III lists means and standard deviations for the various special scales also based on this sample.

K-uncorrected raw scores for Scales 1 through 0 and the conventional validity scales for the three modern samples are shown in Table 1.2. The Mayo Clinic

---

[2]The authors are deeply indebted to Sidney Tuchman, founder of Tuchman Cleaners of Indianapolis, for his unique contribution.

[3]Yet another debt is owed to Major Gary Greenfield for supplying the MMPI records from which the soldier subsample was selected.

TABLE 1.3
Absolute Mean Differences Between the Indiana, MMPI-2,
and Mayo Clinic Norms in Table 1.2

	Female	Male
Clinical Scales		
Indiana vs. MMPI-2	.99	.85
Indiana vs. Mayo Clinic	1.49	1.64
MMPI-2 vs. Mayo Clinic	1.27	.88
Validity Scales		
Indiana vs. MMPI-2	1.33	1.00
Indiana vs. Mayo Clinic	.90	1.33
MMPI-2 vs. Mayo Clinic	.27	.47

norms were provided by the census-matched subsample, presumably the least biased. The slight elevations for the Indiana sample on Scales 4 and 9 could be a result of the absence of respondents over 60 years of age in that sample. The nine items deleted from four different MMPI-2 clinical scales do not appear to have had much effect. Except for the F Scale, on which the Indiana sample is noticeably higher than the other samples, there is a marked concordance among the three samples. Table 1.3 illustrates this agreement by presenting the absolute mean differences in the scores in Table 1.2. The Indiana and MMPI-2 clinical scales average less than one raw score point difference. The Indiana and Mayo Clinic norms are slightly more than one score point apart. The Indiana data for the validity scales tends to be somewhat higher than the other samples, a reflection of the F Scale differences in Table 1.2.

CHAPTER 2
THE VALIDITY SCALES

The creators of the MMPI were aware of the fakability of a verbal inventory. They attempted to develop several validity indicators, internal measures that would point to the individual who was not responding honestly. As it happens, none of these scales is a reliable identifier of the dishonest respondent, though the regular employment of at least one of them—the F Scale—continues. The hardiness of this measure is partly a function of some confusion about the term, *invalidity*. The question is: Valid for what purpose? A scale that elevates when the respondent is badly confused or psychotic suggests that the records may be invalid as personality assessment. Since it assists in diagnosis, it does not indicate that the record is invalid as a diagnostic device.

TRADITIONAL VALIDITY MEASURES

Although less widely known and used than the original MMPI indices, there are three measures that are more effective signallers of the potentially invalid record. Before presenting them, a brief review of the known inadequacies of the earlier scales seems warranted.

Lie Scale

The Lie (L) Scale was constructed by the developers of the MMPI on a completely nonempirical, rational basis. It consists of 15 statements whose context is such that a truthful respondent would be highly likely to respond "True" to every statement. Here are some illustrations of these items.

I do not always tell the truth.
I do not like everyone I know.
I would rather win than lose a game.

The intent of the L Scale is that it should provide "a measure of the degree to which the subject may be attempting to falsify his scores by always choosing the response that places him in the most acceptable light socially" (Hathaway & McKinley, 1951, p. 18). Unfortunately, the gambit is too obvious to anyone of at least average intelligence, a view that is consensually shared by clinicians. An investigation by Lebovits and Ostfeld (1967) not unexpectedly showed that L Scale scores and educational level are negatively correlated.

Yet, almost no one *always* makes the socially acceptable response to the L Scale. Gravitz (1970) collected records of more than 11,000 young adults and found only five L Scale items that came close to the "always" criterion (90% false responses). The deviant (true) response was chosen for four items by more than 50% of the respondents. Hathaway and McKinley (1951) themselves concluded that raw score of 7 on the L Scale was "probably very significant" and would "require interpretation, although not necessarily implying a priori invalidity of the findings" (p. 23).

The L Scale is also insensitive to certain response sets. An individual who endorsed every item would be identified by the maximum L Scale score of 15. But a person who responded "false" to every item would receive a score of 0 and the respondent who alternatingly gave true and false responses would obtain a score of 6, still in the acceptable range according to Hathaway and McKinley.

Occasionally, the L Scale may trap a respondent with his or her best foot forward. The victim is likely to be below the average range of intelligence and with less than a 12th-grade education. But even this isolated case must be examined carefully because high L Scores, although they have little to do with validity of the record, do have meaning and may be interpretable in a different framework. The use of the L Scale as a personality measure is discussed in a subsequent chapter.

F Scale

The F Scale is one of the most misunderstood and misused subsections of the MMPI. It is composed of 64 items that evoked responses in the deviant direction by 10% or less of the segment of the Minnesota standardization sample that was collected prior to 1940. The F Scale was intended as a check on the validity of the record. A high score supposedly indicated that "the other scales are likely to be invalid either because the subject was careless or unable to comprehend the items or because extensive scoring or recording errors were made." A low F score is a "reliable indication that the subject's responses were rational and relatively pertinent" (Hathaway & McKinley, 1951, p. 18). The detection of overreporting or exaggeration of symptoms and distress—so-called faking bad—was not originally mentioned as an intent of the F Scale but it has been widely employed for this purpose. This usage has been endorsed by such MMPI experts as Butcher (1990).

F Scale items were presumably chosen to represent a wide range of content so that a particular bent or pattern by a respondent would not necessarily result in a scale elevation (Meehl & Hathaway, 1946). Simultaneously, item content is thought to be able to identify the faking-bad respondent. Examination of the F Scale suggests that a considerable number of items are not well chosen according to the intent of the scale. Thirteen items—a full 20% of the scale—deal with hallucinations and delusions. Fifteen are found on Scale 8, six on Scale 6, and 10 on the Indiana Severe Reality Distortion scale (see Chapter 5). The correlations between the F Scale and Scales 6, 7, and 8 are substantial (Dahlstrom, et al., 1975). Greene (1991) provides an excellent summary of the investigations demonstrating that elevated F Scale scores are often obtained by severely ill mental patients who are responding truthfully. Graham (1990) goes so far as to recommend that the F scale could be employed as a gross indicator of psychopathology. Greene (1991) concludes that "a specific raw score on the F scale cannot be used to consider profiles as invalid" (p. 110).

With the occasional exception of forensic evaluations, the clinician is unlikely to find that respondents have exaggerated their distress by endorsing items indicative of extreme psychopathology such as delusions and hallucinations. Obvious items dealing with anxiety, depression, and physical symptoms are most often used by respondents wishing to fake bad. There are no more than nine such items in total on the F Scale, a testimony on the other side of the coin to Greene's conclusion.

Finally, over the years, some of the items that were endorsed by no more than 10% of the original MMPI standardization sample have had their appeal altered and would not survive more recent normings. Items 20, 115, 199 and 215 have above 10% endorsement rates in both the Colligan, et al. (1989) norms and the Butcher, et al. (1989) MMPI-2 norms. Item 112 is above the limit for the Colligan et al. females and for both sexes in the Butcher, et al. norms. Similarly, item 185 for the Colligan et al. males and for both sexes in the Butcher, et al. norms. Items 40 and 245 were endorsed by more than 10% of both sexes in the MMPI-2 standardization. Items 14 and 206 are no longer appropriate according to the Colligan, et al. norms. These are among the items dropped in MMPI-2. Items 56, 164 and 252 are over the limit for males in the MMPI-2 standardization data.

In summary, the F Scale is unlikely to identify respondents seeking to exaggerate their pathology. It is not recommended for clinical use though it may be helpful in recognizing subjects who are inappropriate for certain kinds of experiments.

K Scale

The original purpose of this scale was to identify "defensiveness against psychological weakness, and . . . a defensiveness that verges upon deliberate distortion in the direction of making a more 'normal' appearance" (Hathaway &

McKinley, 1951, p. 18). In other words, the respondent who scores high on K is engaging either in denial in the psychodynamic sense or is just plain lying.

The derivation of the K Scale leaves much to be desired. The selection of items was based essentially on a group of 50 psychiatric inpatients all of whom obtained MMPI clinical scale profiles (uncorrected by K, of course) that had no scale above a T-score of 70. A second qualification was that each had an L Scale T-score of at least 60. The idea, of course, was that such individuals, who were identified as seriously ill by reason of hospitalization, were being defensive because of their MMPI records. This assumption has two deficiencies. First, an individual with K-uncorrected T-Scores on clinical scales that are in the 60 to 69 range may be manifesting considerable psychopathology. Second, the L Scale is a poor measure of test-taking defensiveness.

To begin with, a problem arises in the identification of denial as an unconscious mechanism. Denial, like other defense mechanisms, can exist on a psychotic or neurotic level but it can also be an adaptive strategy. Indeed, denial is probably the most common defense mechanism used by normal people (Levitt, 1980b). Is the high K scorer very ill or deliberately lying or symptom-free? Greene (1980) suggested that the K Scale measures normality among normal persons and defensiveness among the maladjusted. The distinction has little empirical backing but in any event, the population to which the respondent belongs is very often unknown. Indeed, the very purpose of the administration of the MMPI may be to determine the population to which the respondent belongs.

Examination of the K Scale items suggests a more lengthy L Scale. It is not difficult to perceive that a normal person who responded truthfully to the best of his/her comprehension could obtain a raw score from 15 to 25, corresponding to T-Scores of 78 and 98 in the Minnesota norms. It also seems evident that an individual who is defending himself/herself against awareness of a negative self-concept could obtain a high score. It also seems possible that individuals with behavior disorders (principal component of the original 50 cases) might obtain a high score through malingering.

In summary, the K Scale does not appear to be useful as a validity measure either on the basis of theoretical considerations or empirical research.

F Minus K Index

Combining the F and K Scales as a validity indicator was proposed by Gough (1950). The idea, of course, is that if F is substantially higher than K, then the respondent is faking bad, trying to exaggerate psychopathology. If the K is so much greater than F, then the respondent was being defensive.

There is no reason to expect that F minus K would be any more effective as a validity indicator than either of its components individually and indeed this seems to be the case. The relevant literature has again been succinctly summed up by Greene (1991). In general, F minus K is at best inconsistent in identifying test-taking attitudes, especially faking bad. It does not function any more effectively in identifying faking bad profiles than does F alone. The union of F and K is no more successful as a validity indicator than either of its components alone and its clinical use is not recommended.

Omitted Items (Qu)

When measurement requires that the subject respond true or false to a fixed number of items, simple common sense indicates that the accuracy of assessment will be impaired if the subject fails to respond to some number of items. Evaluation of the damage as a function of the frequency of omissions is no simple matter.

The number of items to which the subject had failed to respond, Qu, or represented schematically as?, was one of the first ideas about validity that occurred to the developers of the MMPI.

The concept itself was obviously unchallengeable but the number of omitted items that should invalidate a record completely was unknown nor did Hathaway and McKinley have any sound method of making this determination. The use of T-scores made no sense. The Minnesota normative sample omitted a mean of 2.83 items with an SD of 1.5. The omission of a little more than 0.5% of the inventory's items would hardly seem to invalidate a record. Instead, Hathaway and McKinley suggested quite arbitrarily that a Qu above 30 should be viewed with suspicion.

A fair amount of evidence shows that except for a population that is defined by serious deficiency in reading comprehension or by intellectual deficit, no group averages more than a Qu of 5. The mean for the Indiana normative sample was 1.77. While such a finding is of interest, it does not really help in establishing a cut-off point for record invalidity based on omitted items.

A study of Clopton and Neuringer (1979) assessed the impact of omitted items on high-point codes. They found that a little more than 25% of code types were altered by the omission of 30 items. Looking at the other side, more than 40% of the high-point codes were unchanged by the omission of as many as 120 items. The applied significance of this study is unclear but in any event, it has no importance for the clinician who is diagnosing with special scales rather than clinical scales.

Invalidity due to item omission is not a serious problem for the MMPI clinician as long as he/she is aware of the intellectual impact on test validity. It requires about a seventh-grade reading level to be able to complete the MMPI validly (Ward & Ward, 1991). Among those who do not have intellectual problems, clinical experience indicates that less than 1 in 20 will have a Qu of 10 or above. The most commonly omitted items are those about which many people feel uncertain such as "I believe in a life hereafter." Four items that were omitted by more than 10% of the original Minnesota normal group dealt with religious beliefs: 58, 98, 249, and 483 (Dahlstrom et al., 1975). Others deal with circumstances in which the respondent could not have an opinion because of lack of experience such as "When I was a child I liked to play hopscotch" or "I like to read mechanics magazines." Occasionally, items are inadvertently omitted.

While it is true that records are affected by omitted items, they are almost never totally invalidated. Any scale that is elevated despite omissions is all the more significant for that reason. It is more important for the clinician to know which items have been omitted than how many. A cluster of omitted items dealing with the same matter such as family problems or sexual behavior has evident clinical significance. The single omitted item in the case of SV presented in Chapter 6 was a diagnostic clue.

THE NEWER VALIDITY MEASURES

Test-Retest (TR)

Sixteen of the 550 items of the MMPI are duplicated on the first response sheet that was developed for group administration of the inventory. The purpose was to facilitate machine scoring, nothing more. This 566-item form persists even though the replicated 16 items are no longer necessary for scoring purposes. Indeed, it is not at all uncommon to find the MMPI described as an instrument composed of 566 items.[4]

The idea of using the replicated items as a check on the validity of the record was originally suggested by Buechley and Ball (1952). The assumption is that in the valid record, each item in each pair of replicated items will receive the same response. To the extent that responses to the same item are not the same across the 16 pairs, invalidity is suggested. Scores on TR can range from 0 to 16 although Buechley and Ball, for convenience, worked with only 14 pairs of items.

This tactic was later adopted deliberately by Edwards (1959) in the development of his Personal Preference Schedule. He termed the number of agreements among pairs of identical items as a *consistency score*.

Buechley and Ball believed that the major source of invalidity among MMPI records was random responding, probably a function of lack of motivation and unwillingness to bother to read and to try to understand. This does occur among patients and subjects occasionally but clinical experience suggests that two other conditions more often account for elevated TR scores: confusion and poor reading ability or verbal comprehension. Great haste in responding, leading to carelessness, is another possible source of high TR scores.

---

[4]Item duplication has been eliminated in MMPI-2 so that TR is not available in that version of the MMPI.

Bond (1986), on the basis of his research, has proposed that the primary force behind the TR score is simply indecision and thus its utility as a measure of invalidity. is questionable. Indecisiveness is more likely to be a causal factor among Bond's normal college student subjects than it is among patient groups. Bond's data suggest that TR should be applied cautiously with normal subjects who have adequate reading skills.

Carelessness Scale (CLS)

TR is a more effective validity indicator than the F Scale on both logical and empirical grounds. Greene (1978) has pointed out that TR does have one shortcoming. It cannot identify the individual who responds True to every MMPI item or who responds False to every item. Such respondents are rare but they would be missed by TR which would, of course, give them a score of 0.

Greene (1978) devised the Carelessness Scale (CLS) as a validity indicator that did not miss the all-True and all-False respondents. CLS consists of 12 pairs of items, 7 of which should be answered in the same direction on logical grounds and 5 of which should be answered in an opposite direction. Whichever way a thoughtful, clear-headed individual responds to the item, "Most of the time I feel blue," he/she should respond opposite to the item, "I am happy most of the time." Responses to the items, "I am never happier than when I am alone," and "I dislike having people about me," should be the same, whether true or false.

The method of selecting CLS item pairs is somewhat unclear. The MMPI contains many item pairs that should logically elicit responses that are either the same or opposite. On inspection, some of Greene's pairs do not seem well chosen. For example, it appears quite possible to be "afraid to be alone in the dark" and yet not to be "often afraid of the dark." More than one respondent in four in Greene's (1978) three samples gave the deviant response to the item pair, "I am very seldom troubled by constipation," and "I have had no difficulty in starting or holding my bowel movement." The degree of deviancy may be a function of ambiguity of the expression "holding" a bowel movement.

Even if more distinctly discriminating pairs can be found in the MMPI item pool, CLS is a valuable addition to the determination of validity and invalidity. Significantly, it was the model for the True Response Inconsistency Scale and the Variable Response Inconsistency scale, the validity measures of MMPI-2.

Interpreting TR and CLS

TR and CLS are far less likely than the traditional MMPI validity scales to be influenced by severe psychopathology. Their relative subtlety compared to the F and K scales recommends them for clinical use.

Normative TR and CLS data for normal and patient groups are available from a number of sources, e.g., Buechley and Ball (1952), Colligan et al., (1983),

Greene (1978, 1979, 1991) Haymond (1981), Hedlund and Won Cho (cited in Greene, 1991, and Levitt, 1989). The findings are reasonably consistent. Mean scores for normal respondent groups fall between 1.0 and 1.5 on both TR and CLS. For psychiatric patients, the mean score range is from 2.0 to 2.9. Because TR and CLS appear to be getting at different bases for inconsistent responding, it is logical to combine them into a single index. This procedure has been proposed by Nichols, Greene and Schmolck (1989). Their analysis suggests that a TR + CLS score of 8 is the critical determination point. The decision for scores between 7 and 9 is uncertain. Scores below 7 clearly indicate a valid record; invalid records will have a score above 9.

The TR + CLS decision rules recommended by Nichols, et al. (1989) find support from other sources. A TR + CLS score of 8 falls just above a T-score of 70 for the Colligan, et al. (1983) normal subjects and just below T60 for the Hedlund and Won Cho (cited in Greene, 1991) psychiatric patients. A TR + CLS score just above 9 is T70 for the Indiana sample. Scores below 9 were obtained by more than 96% of the normal respondents in the Colligan, et al. (1983) study and by Greene's (1991) normal subjects. Subjects responding with all Trues or all Falses would have a score of 0 on TR but a score of precisely 7 on CLS, thus a score of 7 on TR + CLS.

Mean Elevation (ME)

One of the early research reports on the MMPI (Modlin, 1947) suggested that the average elevation of the nine scales then in existence (including Scale 5 but not Scale 0) could be used as a rough index of psychopathology. Modlin believed that an average elevation of 70 or above (uncorrected for K which was not proposed as a correction until 1948) indicated "major pathology."

No one appears to have taken seriously Modlin's notion that an agglomeration of MMPI clinical scales scores "might be employed as a screening questionnaire or psychosomatic index," and its use as a general index is infrequently reported (e.g., Cernovsky, 1986). The nature of the faking bad profile does, however, suggest a potential use for the average elevation of the clinical scales (ME). Since Scales 5 and 0 are most often uninvolved in the faking bad tactic, the diagnostic capacity of ME is sharpened by basing it on the remaining eight scales.

It is generally agreed that the vast majority of MMPI clinical profiles can be classified as having a high-point pair or high-point code, in the conventional parlance. In the psychiatric patient, the high points may be expected to exceed T70. Other scale elevations might reasonably range from T55 to T69. In a large majority of records, this distribution would yield an ME below T70.

For example, two scales at T75, four scales at T65 and two at T60 would produce an ME of 66. Even if the high-point pair was at T80, ME would be below 68.

However, it is difficult to attain an ME of 75 without diffuse elevation of the clinical scales. For example, even if the high-point pair was at T90, the remaining scales would have to average 70 in order to come out with an ME of 75. Even with three scales at T90, the remaining scales would need to average 66. With three scales at T80, the remaining scales must average 72 in order to yield an ME of 75.

In the Indiana normative sample, ME with K-corrected clinical scales was 58.32 for males and 56.00 for females with corresponding SD's of 5.94 and 6.35. (For K-uncorrected scales, the respective means were 49.02 and 49.01). In these distributions, T75 lies three standard deviations above the mean, an interesting coincidence. Like other validity indicators, the variance of ME has no applied meaning.

Two diagnoses are suggested by a record with an ME of T75 for K-corrected profiles or T70 for uncorrected profiles: 1) an acute psychotic episode, a condition so obvious that psychological evaluation is rarely called for; 2) Borderline Personality Disorder (but see also Chapter 5). Clinical experience dictates that more often, such profiles are a consequence of confusion, inadequate reading comprehension or a faking-bad response set.

CHAPTER 3
SOME USEFUL
SPECIAL SCALES

THE HARRIS AND LINGOES SUBSCALES
OF THE CLINICAL SCALES

Almost from the birth of the MMPI, it has been evident that its clinical scales are multidimensional and that those scales are by no means the only possible effective measuring instruments that could be extracted from the 550 item MMPI pool. An early attempt to capitalize on the multidimensionality were the subscales developed by Harris and Lingoes (1968). They attempted to formulate dimensionally homogeneous subscales from each of the clinical scales using their combined clinical judgment. Apparently, the strategy was a conference technique since no interrater reliabilities were ever reported.

A total of 31 subscales were created from six clinical scales; the items in Scales 1 and 7 did not "lend themselves to classification" according to Harris and Lingoes (1955, rev. 1968). Table 3.1 lists the subscales with their respective descriptions and acronyms.

Subscales derived from Scales 2, 3, 6, and 9 have minimal item overlap except for 2B (D5) which is entirely contained within 2SD (D1). Subscale 4A (Pd4) is the sum of 4SOA (Pd4A) and 4SEA (Pd4B). Subscale 8IPA (Sc2) is a composite of 8COG (Sc2A), 8CON (Sc2B), and 8DIC (Sc2C). The three composite scales are generally not regarded as useful so that the Harris and Lingoes subscales are considered to number 28.

· The Harris and Lingoes scales are employed in clinical situations to some unknown extent. Unfortunately, as Greene (1991) pointed out, research with these

TABLE 3.1
The Harris & Lingoes Subscales of the MMPI Clinical Scales

H & L Designation	H & L Descriptor	Acronym
D1	Subjective Depression	2SD
D2	Psychomotor Retardation	2PR
D3	Physical Malfunctioning	2PM
D4	Mental Dullness	2MD
D5	Brooding	2B
Hy1	Denial of Social Anxiety	3DSA
Hy2	Need for Affection	3NA
Hy3	Lassitude-Malaise	3LM
Hy4	Somatic Complaints	3SC
Hy5	Inhibition of Aggression	3IA
Pd1	Familial Discord	4FD
Pd2	Authority Conflict	4AC
Pd3	Social Imperturbability	4SI
Pd4	Alienation	4A
Pd4a	Social Alienation	4SOA
Pd4b	Self-alienation	4SEA
Pa1	Persecutory Ideas	6PI
Pa2	Poignancy	6P
Pa3	Naiveté	6N
Sc1	Object Loss	8OL
Sc1a	Social Alienation	8SOA
Sc1b	Emotional Alienation	8EA
Sc2	Intrapsychic Autonomy	8IPA
Sc2a	Lack of Ego-Mastery, Cognitive	8COG
Sc2b	Lack of Ego-Mastery, Conative	8CON
Sc2c	Lack of Ego-Mastery, Defect of Inhibition & Control	8DIC
Sc3	Bizarre Sensory Experiences	8BSE
Ma1	Amorality	9AMO
Ma2	Psychomotor Acceleration	9PMA
Ma3	Imperturbability	9IMP
Ma4	Ego Inflation	9EI

scales, especially investigations bearing on validity, is scanty. A statistical study by Lingoes himself (1960) suggested only that factor analyzing the Harris and Lingoes scales results in at least 7 factors and possibly as many as 14. An earlier investigation by Panton (1959) did no more than provide norms for a prison population.

There has been at least one full-scale attempt to examine the criterion validity of the Harris and Lingoes scales (Calvin, 1975). It has a number of methodological shortcomings among which is the sample—all mental patients—that limit inferences that could be drawn from the data. Nevertheless, this study is so rare that it is worthy of commentary.

Calvin set up seven criteria, some of which were clinically based such as diagnosis and patient's attitude toward a significant other as reported by the significant other and by the patient, and the patient's view of his/her reason for admission. Some were less clinical but still hardly objective; the 30-item Nurses Observation Scale for Inpatient Evaluation (NOSIE) and the Gorham Brief Psychiatric Rating Scale (GBPRS) which is based on a psychiatric interview. Neither the NOSIE nor the GBPRS are intended for research and there are no interrater reliabilities in this investigation. Since the NOSIE has 30 items which were used individually by Calvin, there was actually a total of 37 possible criterion measures for any particular Harris and Lingoes scale. The actual number of criteria for a scale varied from as many as 10 to as few as 2, but none was a really firm, objective standard. Calvin himself determined the criteria for each scale, another weakness of this investigation.

Essentially, Calvin found that the Harris and Lingoes subscales on the whole tended to have approximately the same criterion validity as their respective clinical scales. Thus, according to Calvin, "very little is added" to the interpretation of a clinical scale by its Harris and Lingoes subscales. This appears to be true for Scales 2, 6, and 8 which did rather well with their criterion measures. Scales 3, 4, and 9 did more poorly in relating to criteria. The subscales of these clinical scales may be worth noting, although Calvin did not seem to think so. Thus, 3NA (Hy2), 3SC (Hy4), 4FD (Pd1), 4AC (Pd2), and 9IMP (Ma3) were all significantly related to criteria to a greater extent than their respective clinical scales.

Calvin's data are useful in that they reflect some degree of validity for some of the Harris and Lingoes scales. His research, however, does not impinge on a major utility of the Harris and Lingoes scale, i.e., the determination of the cause of a significant elevation of a clinical scale. Because of the multidimensionality of the clinical scales, a respondent may have an elevated score on Scale 3 without symptoms of dissociation; on Scale 4 without being rebellious; on Scale 6 without being paranoid, on Scale 8 without being psychotic, and on Scale 9 without being manic. The subscales assist in determining whether such conclusions are valid. This was the original intent of Harris and Lingoes (1968): the subscales were to be "an aid to profile interpretation." Graham (1978) and Clopton (1979a) have made reference to this original intent and it doubtlessly is the more common utilization of these groupings of items.

What follows are three cases that illustrate this employment of the Harris and Lingoes scales. They were not chosen at random but neither are they atypical. Such cases constitute about 25% of all records, a higher percentage of patient records.

Case D65 has a peak on Scale 6 (Fig. 3.1). The Harris and Lingoes subscales of Scale 6 indicate that this elevation is not due to manifest paranoid ideation: 6PI is not seriously elevated. Also, this respondent endorsed no items on the Indiana Severe Reality Distortion Scale (I-RD) which is composed of all the delusion and hallucination items in the MMPI pool. The other subscales indicate

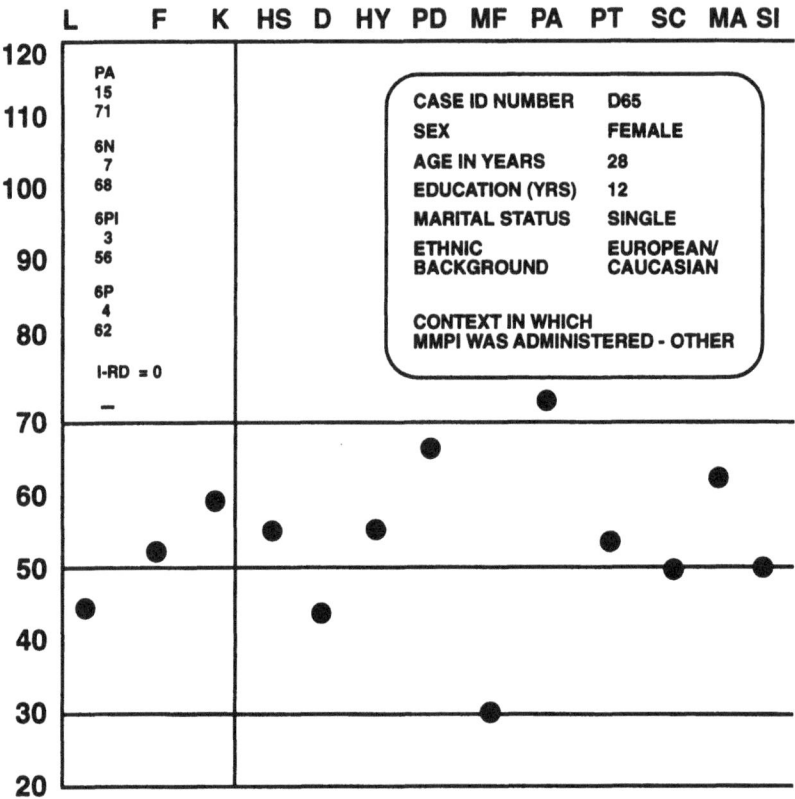

FIG. 3.1. Profile of Case D65.

that the Scale 6 elevation is due primarily to the subject's view of herself as a moral, virtuous individual and one who tends to be somewhat naive (6N-Pa3). The elevation is also a function of some tendency to be hypersensitive (6P-Pa2). These attributes do not add up to a paranoid tendency in the classical sense. One must allow that there are a number of normal women in the community who are naive, somewhat hypersensitive and regard themselves as virtuous.

Case AA38 is a 4-3 but the elevation on the latter scale will stand examination (Fig. 3.2). The Harris and Lingoes subscales of Scale 3 show clearly that an important share of the elevation on that scale is due to 3LM (Hy3) a group of physical symptoms frequently associated with anxiety and depression. Equally importantly, this respondent failed to endorse a single item on the Indiana Dissociative Symptoms Scale (I-DS) which is composed of all the dissociative symptoms in the MMPI pool. In summary, the elevation on Scale 3 does not represent hysterical tendencies in the usual sense but is a function of the fact that this respondent has endorsed a significant number of physical symptom items. Obviously, it is perfectly possible for an individual to have health concerns without being a hysterical personality or even having hysteroid tendencies.

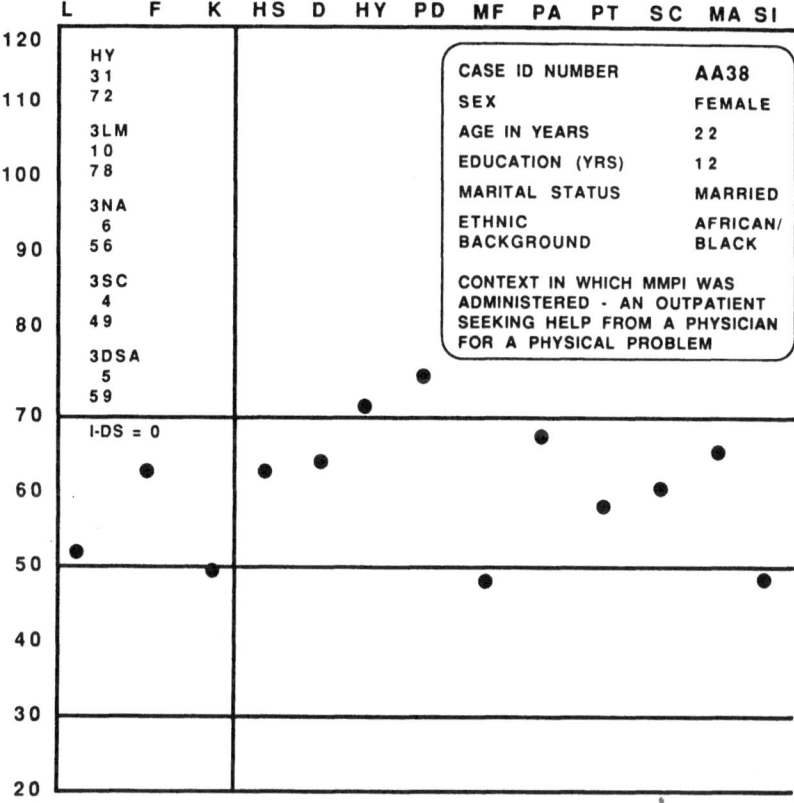

FIG. 3.2. Profile of Case AA38.

Case D54 is the supposedly paradoxical 4-7, more than usually worthy of scrutiny of the subscales (Fig. 3.3). It happens that D54 is socially anxious rather than socially poised—4SI (Pd3) is quite low—her scores are within normal limits on 4SOA (Pd4a), a scale which measures the tendencies to externalize blame, to feel put upon by society and so on, and on 4AC (Pd2), the expression of hostility and rebelliousness. Much of the elevation on Scale 4 is evidently a function of 4SEA (Pd4b) which is composed of a series of depression-like items that describe dissatisfaction with the self rather than the environment, not at all consonant with the conventional interpretation of a high 4.

The tendency for the Harris and Lingoes subscales to follow along with their respective clinical scales has also been reported by Moos and Solomon (1964) and Lebovits, Visotsky, and Ostfeld (1960). As in the Calvin study, there were a few exceptions.

Lebovits et al. administered the MMPI during hallucinogenic experience for a small group of subjects serving as their own control. The subscale changes of interest that occurred were a decrease in 3NA (Hy2) and an increase in 3LM

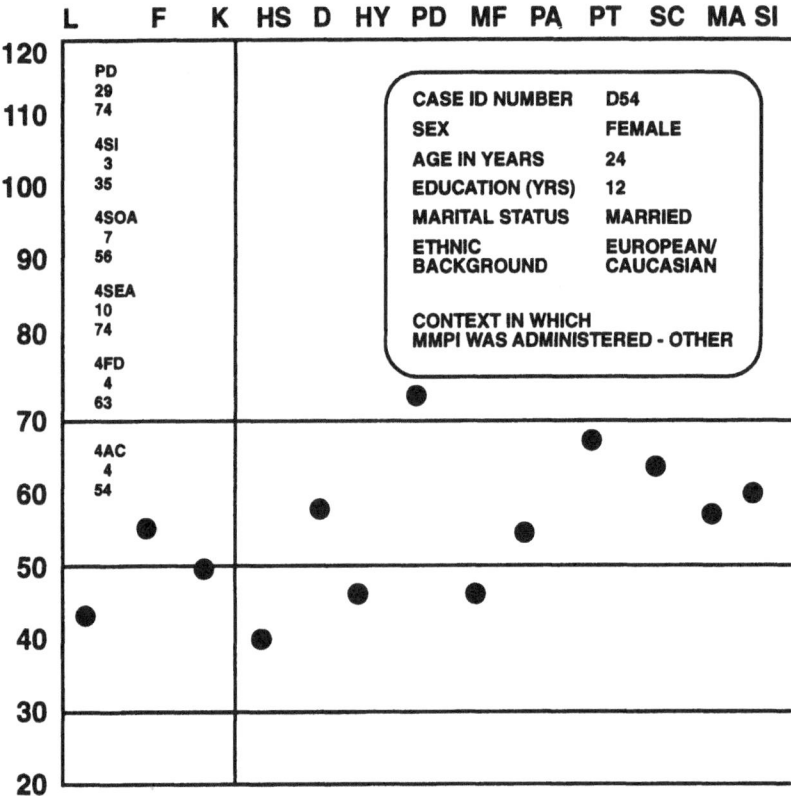

FIG. 3.3. Profile of Case D54.

(Hy3) compared to normal state despite the fact that Scale 3 did not show any interstate difference.

Moos and Solomon compared a group of rheumatoid arthritics with a group of their family members as a control. Again, most of the subscale differences followed clinical scale differences with the notable exception of 8CON (Sc2b) which was significantly elevated in the arthritic group although Scale 8 itself was not. 8CON inversely measures a general motivation, an elan for life, an understandable deficiency in these patients although they are evidently not psychotic.

Individual Harris and Lingoes subscales have occasionally appeared in experimental work. McCreary (1975) compared groups of child molesters with and without a record of prior arrests. The arrested group scored significantly higher on Scale 4 but much of the difference was due to a highly significant difference on 4AC (Pd2). In contrast, 4FD (Pd1) showed hardly even an absolute difference between the two groups. Unfortunately, the remainder of the Harris and Lingoes subscales of Scale 4 are not presented.

3IA (Hy5) failed to distinguish between groups of violent and nonviolent young adult male criminals in a report by Lothstein and Jones (1978). This is one of the Harris and Lingoes subscales that is mislabeled and not useful so this negative finding is not surprising.

Subscale 3IA is one of a number of Harris and Lingoes scales that are mislabeled, have heterogenous item content, have too few items to be directly useful, or have other defects. Table 3.2 presents an analysis of the Harris and Lingoes scales, indicating those that have defects and those that are useful and not useful.

Examination of the item content of the Harris and Lingoes scales discloses that several are clearly heterogenous collections of items that do not appear to belong to the same family. These include 2B (D5), 3IA (Hy5), 8DIC (Sc2c), 8OL (Sc1), and 9EI (Ma4). The titles of 2B, 3IA and 9EI appear to derive from a single item in the subscale. 8DIC (Sc2C) indeed covers what might be broadly termed *defects of inhibition and control*. However, its items deal with a number of individual areas causing loss of control such as dissociation, tension, mania, hypersensitivity, paranoia, and phobia. This heterogeneity makes it all but impossible to interpret a high score on this subscale.

Other subscales also seem to have been mislabeled. This is not particularly surprising. Butcher and Tellegen (1978) once remarked that "new MMPI scales, like many of the old ones, should not be assumed to measure the characteristics suggested by its name or by its author" (p. 623). Harris and Lingoes (1955) themselves cautiously claimed "no particular brief" for their subscale titles and noted that others "would undoubtedly have assigned different names" (p. 1).

Subscales 4SEA (Pd4b) and 8EA (Sc1b) have item homogeneity but are labeled misleadingly. Both are composed primarily of depression items like "Most of the time I feel blue," "I believe I am a condemned person," and "I am happy most of the time (False)." This explains why these two measures had loadings ranging from .70 to .86 on a Depression factor for both sexes in the three patient populations tested by Foerstner (1986) in her factor analytic study of MMPI special scales. These mini-depression scales are inferior to depression scales developed by Wiggins (1966) and by Tryon et al. (Tryon, 1966; Stein, 1968).

Much the same criticism can be made for subscales dealing with health concerns: 2PM (D3), 3LM (Hy3), and 3SC (Hy4). While these serve to separate out the physical symptom aspects of Scales 2 and 3, they contain too few items to be directly useful clinically. Other special scales, notably Wiggins' Poor Health (HEA) and Organic Symptoms (ORG) Scales and the Tryon, Stein, and Chu Body Symptom scale (TSC/B) are more effective measures of health concerns. Similarly, half of the items on 8BSE (Sc3) are duplicated on Wiggins' Organic Symptoms Scale (ORG) which is the superior index of the claim of dissociative/neurological symptoms because of its greater item consistency. On occasion, a smaller health concerns scale elevates while a larger one does not, a circumstance that is worth investigating by direct examination of item content.

TABLE 3.2
Clinical Evaluation of the Harris & Lingoes Subscales

H & L Designation	Acronym	H & L Descriptor	Number of Items	Item Homogeneity	Appropriate Label	Clinical Utility
D1	2SD	Subjective Depression	32	yes	yes	fair
D2	2PR	Psychomotor Retardation	15	yes	yes	good
D3	2PM	Physical Malfunctioning	11	yes	yes	fair
D4	2MD	Mental Dullness	15	yes	yes	good
D5	2B	Brooding	10	no	no	poor
Hy1	3DSA	Denial of Social Anxiety	6	yes	yes	good
Hy2	3NA	Need for Affection	12	yes	yes	good
Hy3	3LM	Lassitude-Malaise	15	yes	yes	fair
Hy4	3SC	Somatic Complaints	17	yes	yes	fair
Hy5	3IA	Inhibition of Aggression	7	no	no	poor
Pd1	4FD	Familial Discord	9	yes	yes	good
Pd2	4AC	Authority Conflict	8	yes	yes	good
Pd3	4SI	Social Imperturbability	12	yes	yes	good
Pd4	4A	Alienation	24	no	no	poor
Pd4a	4SOA	Social Alienation	18	yes	yes	good
Pd4b	4SEA	Self-alienation	15	yes	no	fair
Pa1	6PI	Persecutory Ideas	17	yes	yes	fair
Pa2	6P	Poignancy	9	yes	no	good
Pa3	6N	Naivete	9	yes	yes	good
Sc1	8OL	Object Loss	32	no	no	poor
Sc1a	8SOA	Social Alienation	21	yes	yes	good
Sc1b	8EA	Emotional Alienation	11	yes	no	fair
Sc2	8IPA	Intra-psychic Autonomy	35	no	no	poor
Sc2a	8COG	Lack of Ego-Mastery, Cognitive	10	yes	yes	good
Sc2b	8CON	Lack of Ego-Mastery, Conative	14	yes	yes	good
Sc2c	8DIC	Lack of Ego-Mastery, Defect of Inhibition and Control	11	no	yes	poor
Sc3	8BSE	Bizarre Sensory Experiences	20	yes	yes	fair
Ma1	9AMO	Amorality	6	yes	yes	good
Ma2	9PMA	Psychomotor Acceleration	11	yes	yes	good
Ma3	9IMP	Imperturbability	8	yes	yes	good
Ma4	9EI	Ego Inflation	9	no	no	poor

Fifteen of the Harris and Lingoes subscales have been found to be clinically useful in themselves. They are listed in Table 3.3 along with their clinically based interpretations.

THE WIGGINS CONTENT SCALES

There have been a number of attempts to create new scales by a factor analysis of the MMPI item pool. None has proven as clinically successful as the effort by Wiggins (1966). The explanation of Wiggins' success probably lies in the unconventionality of his methodology.

Any statistical technique that employs samples is subject to error and that includes factor analysis and similar mathematical techniques. This means that in each factor or cluster, there will be some test items that are erroneously assigned to that factor or cluster.

There are at least two procedures for correcting such erroneous assignments and Wiggins employed both. The first is what might be called "expert judgment as to face validity" or what Wiggins termed "intuitive." Wiggins and a colleague examined each factor, identified items which did not appear to fit logically with the factor to which the original analysis had assigned them, and transferred these items to factors with which their content appeared more congruent.

Wiggins also computed correlation coefficients between each item and each of the total factor scores. Those items which had coefficients below .30 or which had higher correlations with any other factor than the one in which it was included were eliminated.

Wiggins does not give the number of items that were manipulated as a function of clinical judgment although the text suggests that the number was considerable. More than 200 items were eliminated as a function of the content analysis. These methodological maneuvers may very well account for the substantial clinical success of the final scales developed by Wiggins.

Fifteen scales resulted from the procedure described thus far. Two of these lacked sufficient internal consistency even after the removal of items and Wiggins decided to abandon them "on the grounds of unpromising homogeneity." The remaining 13 scales have all proven clinically useful.

It should be considered as a tribute to Wiggins' methodology that two of the most recent factor analyses of the MMPI item pool (Johnson, Null, Butcher, & Johnson, 1984; Foerstner, 1986) emerged with approximately the same factors as did Wiggins more than two decades ago.

Clinical Interpretations of the Wiggins Scales

Interpretations of the Wiggins scales have been proposed by Lachar and Alexander (1978) and Graham (1987) as well as by Wiggins himself (1966). Graham also suggested interpretations for low scores on each of the scales. However, the

TABLE 3.3
Clinical Interpretations of Selected Harris & Lingoes Subscales

Subscale	Interpretation
2PR (D2)	High scorers claim to lack sufficient energy to carry on routine activities. When other depression indices are high, a low score on this scale points to a suicide potential.
2MD (D4)	High scorers feel that they are beset by cognitive difficulties: including inability to reason clearly, to make decisions, to think logically. Memory is also impaired.
3DSA (Hy1)	Low scorers tend to be socially maladroit and anxious, shy, to embarrass easily and are generally uncomfortable in social situations. This scale clusters with 4SI (Pd3) and 9IMP (Ma3). High scorers are socially comfortable. Respondents scoring above T70 may be reflecting denial.
3NA (Hy2)	High scorers seek favorable regard by others by adopting a Pollyanna attitude toward society. Scale has a substantial co-fluctuation with 6N.
4SI (Pd3)	See 3DSA.
4AC (Pd2)	High scorers are rebellious and have difficulty accepting standards of behavior that impose responsibilities and interfere with personal gratification. They may be unaware of their angry feelings.
4FD (Pd1)	High scorers reject the family situation and report that it is affectionless, stressful, and lacking in emotional support.
4SOA (Pd4A)	High scorers feel isolated, misunderstood and put upon. They lack a viable social support system and tend to blame others for their problems. This scale co-fluctuates with 8SOA which is interpreted similarly. These respondents are also likely to score high on 4FD, making the claim that family members and intimates fail to provide support.
6P (Pa2)	High scorers regard themselves as hypersensitive. They believe that they can be emotionally injured more easily than others and that they heal less quickly.
6N (Pa3)	High scorers claim to be moral and virtuous; for female respondents, extends to the sexual area. These respondents appear naive and too trusting. They seem to believe that people in general are benign and honest, which justifies their own moral behavior.
8SOA (Sc1A)	See 4SOA. The two scales co-fluctuate markedly despite minimal item overlap.
8COG (Sc2A)	High scorers on this subscale admit to problems similar to those of the high scorer on 2MD: inability to reason, concentrate and remember. However, they believe that their mental processes are not simply obtunded; they have become threateningly strange. Thus, high scorers on 8COG tend to be more disturbed by their cognitive deficits than high scorers on 2MD. The two scales frequently elevate as a pair.
8CON (Sc2B)	High scorers on this scale announce that they are so emotionally upset that they have lost motivation to behave in a constructive or productive fashion. This is often a consequence of cognitive problems that are reflected in high scorers on 2MD and/or 8COG. Tends to co-fluctuate with Work Attitude Scale.
9AMO (Ma1)	High scorers hold to the philosophy that a person is foolish not to take every possible advantage of every situation, usually – but not invariably – short of outright violation of the law. They tend to be somewhat selfish, cynical people who perceive life as an endless series of minor skirmishes in which the person who is not overburdened with scruples is usually victorious. They also believe that most other people share their views.
9PMA (Ma2)	This subscale is a measure of sensation-seeking. High scorers have a high optimal stimulation level, a strong "need for varied, novel, and complex sensations and experience and the willingness to take physical and social risks for the sake of such experience" (Zuckerman, 1979). This subscale is most probably the explanation of why only Scale 9 of the MMPI clinical scales has consistent positive correlations with Zuckerman's Sensation Seeking Scale.
9IMP (Ma3)	See 3DSA.

Wiggins Scales, like most special scales, are unidirectional. Low scores, except for women on the Feminine Interests Scale, have no practical significance.

Table 3.4 presents the interpretations for high scores suggested by Wiggins and Lachar and Alexander. They differ generally in the amount of detail; Lachar and Alexander present a terse summary, Wiggins offers somewhat more detail. Nevertheless, it should be obvious that the two sources are in high agreement concerning interpretation. For each scale, some notes have been added that follow from extended clinical use of these useful scales.

There is a fair number of published reports in the literature using the Wiggins Scales. Only Barron's Ego-Strength Scale and Welsh's A and R Factors appear to have received more attention. By contrast with the latter scales, the reports on the Wiggins Scales are almost unanimously positive, for example, Wiggins, Goldberg, and Applebaum (1971); Taylor, Ptacek, Carithers, Griffin, and Coyne (1972); Payne and Wiggins (1972); Loper, Kammeier, and Hoffmann (1973); Kammeier, Hoffmann, and Loper (1973); Hoffmann, Loper, and Kammeier (1974); Mezzich, Damarin, and Erickson (1974); Boerger (1975); Jarneke and Chambers (1977); Lachar and Alexander (1978); Woodward, Robinowitz, and Penk (1980) and Nichols (1984; 1987).

The Wiggins scales have also proven to be hardy. Most of them survived the restandardization of the MMPI and are still available in MMPI-2 (see discussion in Chapter 7).

THE TRYON, STEIN, AND CHU CLUSTER SCALES

In the 1960s, Tryon and his associates developed a mathematical method for creating independent scales from a large item pool using a special procedure known as cluster analysis which is similar to the usual factor analytic techniques (Tryon, 1966; Stein, 1968). This esoteric statistical technique was applied to 310 MMPI records representing 220 Veterans Administration Hospital inpatients and outpatients and 90 military officers matched with the patients for age and education. The analysis resulted in seven highly reliable clusters that can be considered to be scales for all practical purposes.

The TSC scales have made only rare appearances in research and little is known about their usefulness from experimental data. Stein (1968) reported means on the seven scales for 20 male samples and 13 female samples, most of which had less than 75 subjects. He also reported intercorrelations with the Omnibus Personality Inventory (Heist & Yonge, 1968), the Edwards Personal Preference Schedule (Edwards, 1959) and the Strong Vocational Interest Blank, an earlier version of the Strong-Hansen-Campbell Interest Inventory (Hansen & Campbell, 1985). The samples were small and select: 50 University of California students studying abroad, 50 forestry students, and 50 "public counseling cases" at the University of California Counseling Center. There was a handful of sig-

TABLE 3.4

Interpretations of the Wiggins' Content Scales

	By Wiggins (1966)	By Lachar & Alexander (1978)	Comments
Social Maladjustment (SOC)	High SOC is socially bashful, shy, embarrassed, reticent, self-conscious, and extremely reserved. Low SOC is gregarious, confident, assertive, and relates quickly and easily to others. He is fun loving, the life of a party, a joiner who experiences no difficulty in speaking before a group. This scale would correspond roughly with the popular concept of "introversion–extraversion."	Endorsed item content reflects a lack of social skill and poise, discomfort in social interaction, and resultant inhibition and social isolation. In client populations this lack of social supports may be associated with a negative self-image, feelings of despair or fearfulness, thoughts of suicide, or a defensive orientation characterized by apathy and limited activity or compulsive attention to detail.	Wiggins' interpretation of low scores on SOC does not mesh with clinical experiences. SOC is a one-tailed scale. Also, suicidal ideation is uncommon in high scorers.
Depression (DEP)	High DEP experiences guilt, regret, worry, unhappiness, and a feeling that life has lost its zest. He experiences difficulty in concentrating and has little motivation to pursue things. His self-esteem is low, and he is anxious and apprehensive about the future. He is sensitive to slight, feels misunderstood, and is convinced that he is unworthy and deserves punishment. In short, he is classically depressed.	This individual has admitted to symptoms associated with problematic depression, such as lack of interest in the environment, pessimism, self-criticism, and brooding. In client populations social withdrawal, a negative self-concept, guilt feelings, and a reduced activity level may be suggested.	Wiggins states the case well. But some high DEP persons may simply be screaming loudly for help, not "classically" depressed.
Feminine Interests (FEM)	High FEM admits to liking feminine games, hobbies, and vocations. He denies liking masculine games, hobbies and vocations. Here there is almost complete contamination of content and form that has been noted in other contexts by several writers. Individuals may score high on this scale by presenting themselves as liking many things since this item stem is present in almost all items. They may also score	Inventory responses suggest an interest in pursuits traditionally labeled as feminine and/or dislike of activities stereotyped as masculine. Patient male: In male clients this interest pattern may be associated with an indecisive, passive orientation that has proven to be problematic. Conflict may lead to confusion or self-blame. Evaluation for suicidal ideation or previous attempts is suggested.	It is risky to draw clinical inferences from high FEM scores in males, especially the better educated. Note that both sources refrain from making inferences about sexual preference. But very high scoring females may be protesting too much.

	high by endorsing interests, which, although possibly feminine, are also socially desirable, such as an interest in poetry, dramatics, news of the theater, and artistic pursuits. This has been noted in the case of Wiggins' Sd [Social Desirability] scale. Finally, of course, individuals with a genuine preference for activities that are conceived by our culture as "feminine" will achieve high scores on this scale.	
Authority Conflict (AUT)	High AUT sees life as a jungle and is convinced that others are unscrupulous, dishonest, hypocritical, and motivated only by personal profit. He distrusts others, has little respect for experts, is competitive, and believes that everyone should get away with whatever they can.	Endorsed item content reflects the belief that interpersonal relations are often exploitive in nature. Disregard for principles of ethical conduct and truthfulness is suggested, as well as a tendency to minimize the negative impact of antisocial behavior. In client populations these attitudes may be associated with problematic overassertive and manipulative social relations. Conflict with relatives may result.
Psychoticism (PSY)	High PSY admits to a number of classic psychotic symptoms of a primarily paranoid nature. He admits to hallucinations, strange experiences, loss of control, and classic paranoid delusions of grandeur and persecution. He admits to feelings of unreality, daydreaming, and a sense that things are wrong, while feeling misunderstood by others.	Inventory responses include admission of unusual experiences and beliefs, many of which may include a clearly paranoid component. In client populations this response pattern often suggests an individual who finds comprehension of human motives and behavior difficult and is consequently suspicious of and worried about others. Symptoms associated with a psychotic adjustment, such as ideas of reference, hallucinations, and autistic or disorganized thought, may be present.

Wiggins' interpretation is extreme. It might apply to respondents who score above T70. For scores in the range T58–69, the Lachar-Alexander interpretation is recommended.

Because of the considerable overlap between PSY and alienation scales, sociopathically inclined individuals who are not psychotic may obtain misleading high scores on PSY.

(Continued)

33

TABLE 3.4
(Continued)

	By Wiggins (1966)	By Lachar & Alexander (1978)	Comments
Poor Morale (MOR)	High MOR is lacking in self-confidence, feels that he has failed in life, and is given to despair and a tendency to give up hope. He is extremely sensitive to the feelings and reactions of others and feels misunderstood by them while at the same time being concerned about offending them. He feels useless and is socially suggestible. There is a substantive overlap here between the Depression and Social Maladjustment scales and the Poor Morale scale. The Social Maladjustment scale seems to emphasize a lack of social ascendance and poise, the Depression scale feelings of guilt and apprehension, while the present scale seems to emphasize a lack of self-confidence and hypersensitivity to the opinions of others.	Inventory responses reflect a pervasive lack of confidence in one's abilities and a history of failure, which is related to these perceived limitations. Clients who obtain high Poor Morale elevations may be insecure, despondent, withdrawn, intropunitive, and oversensitive, and may become easily upset by the actions of others.	MOR is primarily an index of self-image, a measure of self-esteem. Of course, correlations with other depression indicators are expected. MOR also has a correlation of .69 with I-SC, a direct measure of negative self-concept.
Religious Fundamentalism (REL)	High scorers on this scale see themselves as religious, church-going people who accept as true a number of fundamentalist religious convictions. They also tend to view their faith as the true one.	Endorsed item content reflects strong religious beliefs and religiously motivated behavior. In client populations this orientation suggests a reduced probability of substance abuse, impulsive behaviors, and conflict with family members. Expression of strong religious beliefs may, at times, reflect a delusional system and associated thought disorder.	The Lachar-Alexander comments on client groups do not negate Wiggins' interpretation. High REL people may be rigid, dogmatic and intolerant, characteristics that can cause interpersonal conflict.

Organic Symptoms (ORG)	High ORG admits to symptoms that are often indicative of organic involvement. These include headaches, nausea, dizziness, loss of mobility and coordination, loss of consciousness, poor concentration and memory, speaking and reading difficulty, disturbing skin sensations, and problems with hearing, smell and muscular control.	This individual has admitted to a variety of sensory, motor, or general somatic concerns that may be related to psychological discomfort and general malaise as well as to reduced effectiveness in completing daily tasks. Clients who obtain high Organic Symptoms elevations may complain of lack of stamina and strength and may present physical symptoms that often indicate emotional conflict, such as problematic headache or back pain.	ORG symptoms *may* indicate organic involvement or they may reflect a dissociative disorder. The scale itself does not distinguish.
Family Problems (FAM)	High FAM feels that he had an unpleasant home life characterized by a lack of love in the family and parents who were unnecessarily critical, nervous, quarrelsome, and quick tempered. Although some items are ambiguous, most are phrased with reference to the parental home rather than the individual's current home.	Inventory responses include admission of pathology in and among family members. A history of poor relationships with parents is suggested, as well as the absence of positive supports in current family interactions, whether with parents, spouse, or extended family. Patient male: In adult male clients admission of family pathology may reflect not only marital conflict but may also suggest intolerant, overactive individuals and a negative self-concept. Drug abuse and other destructive behavior may be associated.	Lachar-Alexander interpretation of high FAM in client males is not supported by clinical experience. Despite item phrasing, most high FAM scorers are referring to the home in which they currently reside.
Manifest Hostility (HOS)	High HOS admits to sadistic impulses and a tendency to be cross, grouchy, competitive, argumentative, uncooperative, and retaliatory in his interpersonal relationships. He is often competitive and socially aggressive.	This individual admits to problems in adjustment related to unmodulated expression of anger, resentment of perceived injustices, need for interpersonal dominance, and limited self-control. In client populations the combination of hostility, moodiness, and impulsivity may be associated with assaultive or other antisocial or violent behavior.	HOS is an excellent measure of experienced anger but "sadistic" is a bit extreme.

(Continued)

TABLE 3.4
(Continued)

	By Wiggins (1966)	By Lachar & Alexander (1978)	Comments
Phobias (PHO)	High PHO has admitted to a number of fears, many of them of the classically phobic variety such as heights, dark, closed spaces, etc.	This individual admits to a variety of fears and appears to be significantly uncomfortable in many situations. Clients who obtain high PHO elevations are viewed as more anxious, tremulous, worrisome, and phobic than most patients. Depression and social withdrawal may also be indicated.	Almost half of the items in PHO do not refer to phobias directly. Scores as high as T60 may be obtained by individuals who are not phobic.
Hypomania (HYP)	High HYP is characterized by feelings of excitement, well-being, restlessness, and tension.	This individual's self-description suggests a fast personal tempo characterized by enthusiasm, cheerfulness, and perhaps irritability or emotional lability. Clients who obtain high Hypomania elevations are often described as immature, hyperactive, excitable, agitated, and restless. They are unlikely to respond intropunitively to conflict and may manipulate others to reach their goals.	Wiggins' interpretation is valid for scores in the range of T60-69. Above T70, the Lachar-Alexander interpretation applies, whether the respondent is a client or not.
Poor Health (HEA)	High HEA is concerned about his health and has admitted to a variety of gastrointestinal complaints centering around an upset stomach and difficulty in elimination.	A significant number of physical complaints are reflected by item endorsement centering mainly around the digestive system. Individuals who obtain high Poor Health elevations are often considerably worried about their health. Cardiac and pulmonary complaints are also occasionally reported.	

Source: Wiggins (1966) and Lachar & Alexander (1978). Reprinted by permission of the copyright holder, the American Psychological Association, and the authors.

nificant correlation coefficients but their bearing on the validity of the various TSC scales is unclear.

Boerger (1975) obtained TSC scale scores along with 18 other MMPI special scales scores from two samples comprising 679 psychiatric inpatients. Sixty-three criterion variables were employed in a vast fishing expedition similar to the effort by Calvin (1975) previously described. Like Calvin, Boerger used the NOSIE and the GBPRS among his criterion measures.

Boerger analyzed his data by comparing mean scores for the highest scoring 25% of the sample on each scale with the remainder of the sample, and the lowest scoring 25% with the remainder of the sample. A rationale for the use of this weak method of analysis is not offered. A correlational technique would seem to be more appropriate and potentially revealing. Even a comparison of the upper and lower quartiles would make more sense.

A bit less than 15% of all the mean comparisons for the TSC scales were significant at the 10% level—a coincidence that has a suspicious smell of chance. Boerger's criterion, however, was significance in both samples; his reasoning was that $.10 \times .10 = .01$. A very much smaller number of comparisons reached Boerger's criterion. Since this was an inpatient group, TSC/S, TSC/D and TSC/A did much better than TSC/I, TSC/B, and TSC/R and there is a suggestion of support for validity for the former threesome. But this consideration applies only to the TSC scales as measures of psychopathology. The Boerger data, at best inconclusive, do not bear on the utility of the TSC scales as personality measures.

Clinically, all the TSC scales except TSC/A have been found to be useful measures. Table 3.5 provides the clinically based interpretations of these six scales.

THE INDIANA RATIONAL SCALES

The continued use of Lushene's program over the years, with several revisions, at the Indiana University Medical Center led to the realization that existing MMPI scales did not successfully tap certain important areas. Psychologists at the Medical Center who were involved with Lushene's program decided to create some new scales covering the uncovered areas. The technique was face validity following from the title of the scale, a rational rather than an empirical process. This method has been demonstrated to be the most effective procedure for selecting items for inventory scales (Ashton & Goldberg, 1973; Jackson, 1975; Gynther, Burkhart, & Hovanitz, 1979).

Seven scales were developed by means of expert judgments. Three judges[5] determined the items for four of the scales. Only those items were included that were agreed upon by all three judges.

---

[5]The judges were Frank J. Connolly, Dr. Wm. George McAdoo and the senior author, who organized the Multiphasic Data Analysis Corporation in 1977. MDAC was the source of many of the records that furnished the basis for clinical interpretation of special scales in this book. The Indiana scales were unofficially known as MDAC scales originally.

TABLE 3.5
Interpretation of the Tryon, Stein, and Chu Scales

TSC Scale	Interpretation
Body Symptoms	High scorers are anxious about their physical health; they claim to have a variety of physical symptoms of the type commonly associated with anxiety and depression such as pains, easy fatigability, feelings of weakness and minor gastrointestinal complaints.
Depression	High scorers are depressed, unhappy, brood a great deal, and feel under chronic tension. They lack energy and feel useless, incapable and guilty.
Resentment	High scorers tend to express hostility in a typically adolescent pattern; they tend to feel imposed upon and denigrated and are likely to be impatient and irritable.
Social Introversion	High scorers are shy, socially uncomfortable, easily embarrassed and tend to withdraw when faced by stress, especially in situations involving interpersonal relations.
Suspicion	High scorers are likely to be cynical and opportunistic and to mistrust the sincerity and benignity of the motivations of others. They may have a sociopathic orientation but are not necessarily paranoid in the classical sense. Low scorers tend to be naive and suggestible and are relatively easily manipulated.
Tension	High scorers are anxiety-prone, claim to worry chronically, tend to become tense easily.

Severe Reality Distortions (I-RD) (18 items)
Dissociative Symptoms (I-DS) (8 items)
Obsessive-Compulsiveness (I-OC) (9 items)
Sex Problems (I-SP) (14 items)[6]

A fourth judge was added for the creation of two additional scales:[7]

Self-Concept (I-SC) (14 items)
Dependency (I-De) (9 items)

Only those items were included that were agreed upon by three of the four judges. A seventh scale, Dominance (I-Do) (17 items), was developed independently by the author.

Since the judges, as clinical psychologists, shared a common educational background as well as a common workplace, the concepts used as scale titles were not defined. The only instruction was that every scale item should be manifestly face valid, requiring little or no inference to justify its inclusion in the scale. There were two special conditions. It was understood beforehand by the judges that only items dealing directly with hallucinations and delusions should be selected for I-RD. In selecting items for I-De, the judges began with the 54 items in the Navran Dependency Scale (Navran, 1954).

---

[6]Only 12 items are scored for female respondents. See Appendix I.
[7]The fourth judge was Dr. Richard J. Lawlor.

Severe Reality Distortion Scale

Diagnosing a psychosis with the MMPI or any verbal inventory is always risky (see, for example, Affleck & Garfield, 1960). To begin with, the intensity or degree of disturbance reflected in items is not necessarily an accurate indicator. There are a number of explanations for high-ranging, psychotic-like clinical profiles on the MMPI. Such profiles are obtained by respondents "faking bad" for whatever reason, severe obsessive–compulsives, and individuals lacking sufficient reading comprehension. Diagnosis by critical items taken individually is also a method with minimal reliability.

As Koss, Butcher, and Hoffman (1976) noted:

> Single items are risky sources of important clinical interpretation compared to scales of multiple items. A patient can misread, misinterpret, or mismark a response to a single item and invalidate the item as a correct sample of behavior. (p. 923)

Evidence comes from a small investigation conducted at Indiana University Hospitals. The MMPI was administered to 20 consecutive patients admitted to the hospital in the summer of 1979. Records were scored for a selected set of 46 critical items of which only 11 overlapped with the F Scale. A total of 181 critical items were endorsed by all patients, a mean of just a bit more than nine per patient. One or 2 days after, each patient was interviewed concerning the critical items. Thirty percent of the endorsements—nearly three per patient on the average—were denied. The patients insisted that they had never endorsed about two out of three of the denied items and had misinterpreted one of three. Fifty-two percent of the items dealing with severe reality distortions, such as hallucinations and delusions, were denied or misinterpreted.

A reasonable conception is that the most reliable method of diagnosing psychosis with the MMPI is by means of a scale that encompasses all items for which an endorsement appears to indicate the existence or recent existence of an hallucination or delusion. There are 18 such items on the MMPI; they constitute I-RD.

Clinical experience indicates that I-RD is, indeed, the most reliable psychotic indicator that can be formed from the MMPI pool. It is superior for this purpose to the six signs proposed by Peterson (1954), the ratio developed by Sines and Silver (1963) or Wiggins' Psychoticism Scale, although the latter is a useful measure of the intensity of emotional disturbance.

Not all high scorers on I-RD are psychotic, but the probability of psychosis is sufficiently high so that attention should be called to the possibility in the clinical report.

Dissociative Symptoms Scale

I-DS consists of eight items for which the deviant response clearly suggests the presence of a dissociative symptom. Hysteroid personalities are likely to have elevations of T60; individuals scoring at T70 or above are usually the victims of severe dissociative disorders except when I-RD is also significantly elevated. In such instances, the dissociative symptoms are part of the psychosis complex. A recent study (Nash, Hulsey, Sexton, Harralson, & Lambert, 1993) found that I-DS successfully differentiated among four groups of women grouped on the basis of sexual abuse-nonabuse as children.

Obsessive–Compulsiveness Scale

I-OC consists of nine statements. Three are obvious compulsive rituals, three describe obsessive rumination and three are indicative of obsessive persistence and caution. Individuals with obsessional traits or even obsessive–compulsive personalities rarely score high on I-OC. A high score on I-OC indicates severe obsessive–compulsive disorder, either as neurosis or as an aspect of a psychotic disorder.

Self-Concept

I-SC measures the extent to which the individual has a negative self-image. Its 12 items contain only three that are found on Scale 2. Individuals scoring high on this scale are low in self-esteem and self-confidence, and regard themselves as relatively incapable and generally unattractive.

Sex Problems

I-SP was originally composed of 15 items. Experience with clinical use of this scale indicated that one item should be dropped and that two others should be scored only for male respondents. Accordingly, the current version has 14 items that are scored for the male respondent and 12 for the female respondent. Individuals scoring high on I-SP may have any one of a variety of sexual dysfunctions. The scale is not useful in diagnosing paraphilias or sexual deviations, however.

Dependency

The 10 items in I-De were chosen from the 57 proposed as a dependency measure by Navran (1954). I-De is somewhat lacking in effective psychometric properties, notably the distribution of scores tends to be limited. However, I-De is still useful when interpreted together with the Indiana Dominance Scale (I-Do).

Dominance

The 17 items of this scale describe an individual who has strong views that are strongly defended, regards himself/herself as relatively independent of the views of others, is outspoken and self-confident. Like I-De, scores on I-Do appear to have a restricted range. Nevertheless, this scale can be usefully interpreted in conjunction with I-De.

The following rules have been found to be effective:

- Dependent individuals will have a score on I-De that is at least T50 and a score on I-Do that is below T40. Males conforming to this pattern tend to be more noticeably passive, submissive and easily manipulated than women with the pattern.
- Individuals with a need to dominate others will have a score on I-Do that is at least T50 and a score on I-De that does not reach as high as T40. Such individuals are not necessarily dominant. The scales describe a need; whether the individual is successful in satisfying this need or not is not reflected in the scale scores.
- Individuals whose scores do not fall into one of the two previous patterns can be said to be unremarkable with respect to their dependency and dominance needs.

SOME SPECIAL SCALES

Among the Harris and Lingoes subscales, the Wiggins Content Scales, the Tryon, Stein, and Chu Cluster Scales and Indiana Scales, there are some 43 clinically proven measures covering a wide range of symptoms and traits. This group of scales substantially exceeds the diagnostic capacity of the conventional clinical scales. But there are a number of other scales of proven utility that should be included in the armamentarium of the clinician who makes use of special scales.

The Pepper and Strong Altruism Scale (5C)

In an unpublished report, Pepper and Strong (1958) proposed a five subscale breakdown of the MMPI Scale 5 (Masculinity–Femininity). The Pepper and Strong breakdown of Scale 5 resulted in the following subscales:

Denial of Masculine Occupational Interests (5DMO)
Feminine Occupational Interests (5FOI)
Personal and Emotional Sensitivity (5PES)
Sexual Identification (5SI)
Altruism (5A)

The Pepper and Strong scales are probably superior to the breakdown of Scale 5 suggested by Serkownek (Schuerger, Foerstner, Serkownek, & Ritz, 1987). However, clinical experience indicates that only one of the Pepper and Strong scales is independently useful.

5DMO and 5FOI are neatly encompassed in Wiggins Feminine Interests Scale. 5PES is redundant with the Harris and Lingoes Poignancy Scale (6P). 5SI is mislabeled and is not useful.

Individuals scoring high on 5A endorse traditional American cultural values like honesty, candor, and fair play. They tend to be somewhat unsophisticated; scale scores have moderate positive correlations with 3NA and 6N and are also positively related to Lie Scale scores. "Altruism" hardly seems to be a good descriptor for this scale, although no doubt high scorers would agree that generosity and selflessness are virtues. *Conventionality* appears to be a more appropriate label, thus 5C.

Cynicism Scale (E/Cy)

One of the several factor analyses of the MMPI pool was carried out by Eichman, originally with female inpatients (Eichman, 1961) and later extended to male inpatients (Eichman, 1962). In both investigations, four factors were identified. The first three were labeled Anxiety, Repression, and Somatization. Eichman was uncertain about the label for Factor IV. At first, he decided to call it Acting-Out on the grounds that the clinical loadings suggested that the factor might be measuring either psychoticism or sociopathy. After collecting the male data, Eichman decided to call Factor IV Unconventionality on the grounds that the item content "carries the flavor of unconventional, impulsive, and perhaps bizarre behavior . . ." (p. 367). He allowed, however, that "the meaning of a high IV score in the normal population is important but remains to be done" (p. 380).

Factor IV contains 20 items in the scale for males and 20 for females with 14 items in common. Examination of the item content certainly would not lead to an inference that the appropriate title for the scale is Unconventionality. A high scorer on Factor IV would be no more likely to be unconventional than a high scorer on any number of other sets of 20 MMPI items. The content examination suggests that a majority of the items for both males and females appear to be tapping a characteristic that might best be labeled *cynicism*. Most of the remaining items, though they do not appear to be measuring cynicism directly, are at least not sharply incompatible with this assessment.

E/Cy tends to elevate along with alienation and suspicion scales, as in the records of sociopathically inclined individuals, much as might be expected (see Chapter 5). It has minimal or no item overlap with scales measuring alienation and suspicion and thus is a distinct contribution to the measurement of personality tendencies.

The Cook and Medley Hostility Scale (Ho)

Ho was originally part of a group of 77 items chosen because they discriminated between school teachers scoring high and low on the Minnesota Teacher Attitude Inventory. Five clinical psychologists then selected the final 50-item version of Ho on the basis of "substantial agreement," which is not defined by Cook and Medley (1954).

Ho is one of the few special scales that has been used in published research and it has given rise to some interesting findings. Jurjevich (1963) found that Ho did a better job of relating to the subscales of the Buss–Durkee Hostility–Guilt Index (Buss & Durkee, 1957) than five other item sets derived from the MMPI including Scales 4 and 6. McGee (1954) found that Ho had low but significant correlations with a word association test and a picture sorting test designed to measure hostility. Shaw and Grubb (1958) reported that underachieving male high school sophomores obtained a higher Ho score than achievers, according to hypothesis. Ho also correlated .79 for females and .85 for males with the Hostility Scale of the Guilford-Zimmerman Temperament Survey. However, Megargee and Mendelsohn (1962) reported that Ho, like 11 other MMPI measures related to hostility, failed to discriminate among three groups classified as extremely assaultive criminals, moderately assaultive criminals and nonassaultive criminals, and a group of noncriminals.

More recently, Ho has entered the health psychology field. Williams et al. (1980) found a significant relationship between scores on Ho and the severity of coronary artery disease in a sample of more than 400 patients who underwent coronary angiography. In fact, Ho scores predicted the severity more efficiently than interview-based ratings of Type A behavior. Smith and Frohm (1985), in a questionnaire study, reported that high Ho scorers were beset by the combination of a less satisfactory social support system and more frequent irritating events making for what the authors characterize as "a distinctly negative psychosocial risk factor profile" (p. 514).

Barefoot, Dahlstrom, and Williams (1983) and Shekelle, Gale, Ostfeld, and Paul (1983) reported that Ho was a predictor of the incidence of heart attacks and cardiac deaths over extended periods of time.

Spielberger, Jacobs, Russell, and Crane (1983) found a significant correlation that averaged around .50 between Ho and the trait form of the State-Trait Anger Scale. A significant correlation was also reported between Ho and estimated potential for hostility based on interviews by Dembroski, MacDougall, Williams, Haney, and Blumenthal (1985).

On the whole, the various field studies of Ho are strong testimony to its validity but do not necessarily support the Cook and Medley choice of a scale designation. There is no firm, independently verified theoretical structure from which one could predict that high school underachievers would be more hostile than achievers or that individuals developing coronary artery disease are more given to trait hostility than those who do not.

A factor analysis of the MMPI item pool (Johnson, Null, Butcher, & Johnson, 1984) resulted in a set of factors that included a 20-item factor labeled by expert decision, Cynicism. Sixteen of those 20 items are common to Ho. Another factor analysis of the MMPI pool (Costa, Zonderman, McCrae, & Williams, 1985) also resulted in a Cynicism factor with 22 items in common with Ho.

The cynicism content of Ho is so marked that Smith and Frohm (1985) suggest that the scale should be called Cynical Hostility. Their statement of high scores on Ho dovetails neatly with clinical experience:

> High Ho scorers are prone to anger and are suspicious and resentful of others. Though not necessarily more likely to report physical aggressiveness, they view others with distrust and are likely to be vigilant, calculating, and manipulative in their social interactions. . . . These persons are likely to become dysphoric, to feel isolated and dissatisfied with their social supports, and to experience more frequent and subjectively severe daily irritants. (p. 516)

Overcontrolled Hostility Scale (OH)

Several reasonably careful investigations arrived at the interesting conclusion that institutionalized criminals convicted of violent crimes tend to score lower on measures of aggression and higher on measures of control than do nonassaultive criminals and normal men (Megargee & Mendelsohn, 1962; Blackburn, 1968). This curious finding led Megargee (1966) to the conclusion that assaultive criminals come in two types: undercontrolled and overcontrolled. Accordingly, he set about devising a scale for the measurement of hostility in the overcontrolled person (Megargee, Cook, & Mendelsohn, 1967).

The 31 items of the OH scale are based on MMPI records of four groups: extremely assaultive men convicted of murder, assault with a deadly weapon, and so on; moderately assaultive men convicted of no more than battery; criminals convicted for crimes other than violence, and normal men. Item analyses resulted in a 55 item scale that differentiated the assaultive from non-assaultive prisoners. However, there was considerable overlap between the distributions. The scale was refined by cross-validation on a new sample of incarcerated offenders. The result was a 31-item scale that not only discriminated assaultive from nonassaultive prisoners but also distinguished between a group of violent criminals classified as overcontrolled and undercontrolled through expert clinical judgment on the basis of examination of prison records.

Megargee et al. (1967) assert that the scale measures simultaneously "two personality constructs which are not normally found together, impulse control and hostile alienation." Thus, they believe that high scorers on OH have serious conflict between strong aggressive impulses and perhaps strong inhibitions against the expression of aggression. The net consequence is that the hostile impulses are chronically restrained until they mount to a critical intensity at which point the individual is likely to explode into a sudden act of extreme violence or perhaps psychosis.

The OH scale is one of the few that has been subjected to a considerable amount of postdevelopment investigation. Most of the reported investigations support the validity of OH in one way or another (deGroot & Adamson, 1973; Blackburn, 1972; Fredericksen, 1975; Haven, 1972; Lane & Kling, 1979; Megargee, 1969; Vanderbeck, 1973; White, 1970, 1975; White, McAdoo, & Megargee, 1973). Those investigations in which positive findings for validity were not obtained used unsound methodology: administering OH in isolation instead of within the entire MMPI (Lester, Perdue, Brookhart, 1974; Mallory & Walker, 1972; Rawlings, 1973) or using criterion groups that were contaminated by racial bias (Fisher, 1970).

OH was developed with male prisoners and almost all of the subsequent work has tested male samples. The single investigation which included female murderers reported some evidence that OH could also apply to women (Sutker & Allain, 1979). However, the evidence for validity is not strong and this is one of the few studies that did not support the ability of OH to discriminate among male prisoners.

The clinical utility of OH would be very restricted if it were applicable only to samples of incarcerated criminals. As it happens, the value of this interesting set of items ranges considerably beyond such limitations. Clinically, we find that noncriminal male and female high scorers on OH behave very much in accordance with the theoretical position of Megargee et al. (1967). They appear to have strong inhibitions against the expression of aggression and characteristically deny hostile feelings, usually obtaining low scores on such scales as HOS. They are considered to be quiet, passive, and unassuming. They are also given to aperiodic rage reactions in which they may or may not attack others or destroy property. They are rarely murderers.

Table 3.6 provides MMPI data on a single, white, unemployed male, age 34 with an eighth-grade education. He was referred by the police after 20 arrests for public intoxication which often included violent behavior.

Scores on manifest hostility (AUT and HOS) were quite low. The respondent's score on the TSC Resentment scale is within limits. His OH score is very high and his AMac indicates that he is probably an alcoholic or drug abuser or is at risk for becoming one or the other (see discussion of AMac in Chapter 4).

An appropriate interpretation would be that this individual typically represses hostility, that he is able to obtain release from the emotional strain of denial and repression by becoming disinhibited with alcohol at which times he acts out aggressively.

Assertiveness

Occasionally, a special scale constructor using the contrasting groups technique will fail in the designed purpose but will succeed serendipitously in creating a new useful scale. The unsuccessful aim of an investigation by Ohlson and Wilson (1974) was to distinguish homosexual from heterosexual females using an in-

TABLE 3.6

A Case Illustrating the Use of Special Scales to Identify Overcontrolled Hostility*

AUT	HOS	TSC/R	OH	AMac
39	39	49	73	26

*The AMac datum is a raw score; all others are T-scores. The patient is male, white, single, age 34, unemployed.

ventory composed of MMPI items. The contrasting groups were a sample of lesbians who were active in the gay liberation movement and a carefully matched sample of heterosexual females.

All raw score differences between the two groups on the clinical scales and the conventional validity scales were small although the heterosexual group scored significantly higher on Scales 1, 3, and 7. Fifty-six items differentiated the two groups at the 2% level or beyond; of course, two of these were items No. 69 "I am strongly attracted to members of my own sex," and No. 430 "I am attracted by members of the opposite sex."

Unfortunately, Ohlson and Wilson do not give mean scores on the 56 items for their contrasting groups but clinical experience suggests that while the lesbian group doubtlessly scored higher than the heterosexual sample, there was considerable overlap of the distributions. Using the items diagnostically would result in a spate of false positives. The 56 items as a scale are not recommended for identifying homosexual females.

Examination of the content of the items suggests that they tap not lesbianism but a correlative characteristic of members of the gay liberation movement—assertiveness. Assertiveness is used in this sense as a non-noxious behavior apart from aggression (e.g., Hollandsworth, 1977; Hollandsworth & Wall, 1977). Twenty percent of the items deal directly with this characteristic; most of these were referred to as representing a "masculine orientation" by Ohlson and Wilson. Another large group of items deal with physical health and emotional adjustment which are not unreasonably associated with assertiveness in women. About 10% of the items are stereotypically feminine characteristics that are likely not to be found in assertive women.

Clinical experience suggests that an Assertiveness scale (Astvn) for women composed of the Ohlson–Wilson items except for Nos. 69 and 430, has assessment value.

THE OBVIOUS–SUBTLE DISTINCTION APPLIED TO SPECIAL SCALES

As has already been pointed out, an early demonstration of the multidimensionality of MMPI clinical scales was the separation of items into obvious and subtle categories. In principle, an obvious item is one for which the significance of a true or false response should be manifest to most respondents. Few adults would have difficulty comprehending the meaning of endorsement of items like "I work under a great deal of tension," or "I have had very peculiar and strange experiences." On the other hand, the assessment meaning of endorsing an item like "At times I feel that I can make up my mind with unusually great ease," or denying "I like to talk about sex" would not be understood by most respondents.

Wiener and Harmon

The original classification of MMPI items as obvious or subtle was the work of Wiener and Harmon (1964), later published under Wiener's name (Wiener, 1948, 1956). Wiener and Harmon essentially used two methods of distinguishing items. All items on the F Scale and on Scales 1, 7, 8 were automatically assigned to the obvious category on the grounds that they measured psychopathology, presumably directly, although this is not specifically stated. Most of the remaining items were categorized by the authors' "pooled judgments"; the procedure is not detailed any further.

It is plain that by "obvious" Wiener and Harmon meant that the item clearly described a bit of psychopathology on a particular clinical scale. This point is indicated by the fact that there are eight items keyed in the same direction that were designated as obvious on one scale and subtle on another. For example, the item "My hardest battles are with myself" (True) is classified as obvious on Scale 7 and subtle on Scale 4.

The notion that an item can be obvious on one scale and subtle on another is not sensible. It hints at the ridiculous possibility that respondents not only can determine the significance of endorsement or denial of the item but can also determine to which clinical scale or scales the item belongs. It makes more sense simply to judge whether or not the average respondent could tell whether or not a response admits to psychopathology.

Wiener (1948, 1956) reported early that the obvious sets of items were not statistically related to the subtle items. The average intercorrelation was −.50. The highest positive correlation was only .24 (Scale 9). He also reported that the obvious items alone differentiated successful from unsuccessful students and job trainees while the total scores on the clinical scales did not differentiate.

These two findings have been reported from a number of sources over the years, most recently by Wrobel and Lachar (1982). The incapacity of the subtle items of the MMPI is a telling argument against the use of the clinical scales and in favor of a battery of special scales.

Another Approach to the Obvious–Subtle Distinction

All that we know about psychological measurement suggests that the approach to the obvious–subtle distinction used by Wiener and Harmon is too simplistic. Few phenomena of human life are naturally dichotomous; there should be degrees of obviousness and subtlety. Indeed, this seems to be the case. One could easily dispute the assignment of an item like "My hands and feet are usually warm enough," or "I loved my father," to the obvious category, or "At times I have very much wanted to leave home," or "My hardest battles are with myself," to the subtle category. These items, like many others, appear to be not quite obvious and not quite subtle.

Christian, Burkhart, and Gynther (1978) approached the obvious–subtle distinction from the position that obvious and subtle are ends of a dimension rather than merely a dichotomy. They asked a large group of college students to make estimates on a 5-point scale ranging from 1 (most subtle) to 5 (most obvious). The mean estimate per item was then computed. In this procedure, "I have a good appetite," has a mean rating of 2.91 and "My hands and feet are usually warm enough," has a mean rating of 2.67, both on the subtle side of the scale. On the other side of the Wiener and Harmon ledger, "At times I have very much wanted to leave home," received a mean rating of 3.46 and "At times I feel like picking a fist fight with someone," obtained a mean rating of 3.74. Both are at the obvious end of the scale.

The reference group used by Christian et al. is perhaps not the most appropriate one but it does represent a population of potential subjects for the application of the MMPI. More importantly, it provides a more refined statement of obviousness and subtlety than a dichotomous system.

Table 3.7 gives a comparison of the proportions of subtle items assigned to the F Scale and the eight clinical scales compared with the proportions of items that had mean ratings below 2.5, the midpoint of the 5-point scale according to the raters employed by Christian et al.

In general, Wiener and Harmon found more subtle items than did the raters of Christian et al., 23% against 17.7%. Wiener and Harmon made no judgments for the F Scale and for Scales 1, 7, and 8, deciding that all items in those scales were obvious. Computing only for the remaining five scales, the mean subtle percent by Wiener and Harmon is 57, by Christian et al. only 30. Nevertheless, it appears that Wiener and Harmon were not far afield when they decided to deal only with five scales. The mean subtle percentage for Scales 1, 7, and 8 and the F Scale according to the raters of Christian et al. is only 4.5.

The difference in assignments between Wiener and Harmon and the Christian et al. raters may be partly a function of improved diagnostic skills over a 30-year period. It is also clearly due to the effect of the 5-point as opposed to the 2-point categorization. Wiener and Harmon apparently assigned more of the doubtful items to the subtle category, for whatever reasons.

Using the Obvious–Subtle Ratings.   Obvious–subtle ratings based on the work of Christian et al. were computed for each special scale described in this volume by averaging the ratings of its items. These means are presented along with their respective scales in Appendix IV.

TABLE 3.7
A Comparison of Subtlety on the MMPI Clinical Scales

Scale		Percent Subtle Items	
		Wiener & Harmon	Christian et al.*
F		0	6
Hs	(1)	0	9
D	(2)	33	30
Hy	(3)	47	37
Pd	(4)	43	22
Pa	(6)	43	23
Pt	(7)	0	2
Sc	(8)	0	1
Ma	(9)	50	35
Overall		23	17.7

*Items having a mean rating of 2.5 or less.

The common practice among high-point code typologists is to discard the "faking bad" record as invalid and therefore uninterpretable. Even when the respondent is indeed "faking bad," there will be some scales among the special scales that may still be validly interpreted. Exaggeration of psychopathology is almost always accomplished by endorsements of obvious items. The point appears uncontestable; how could a respondent fake if he/she was unable to fathom the significance of a true or false response to the item? The empirical demonstration of this axiom by Burkhart, Christian, and Gynther (1978) is almost gratuitous.

In general, scales that have a definite obvious quality such as PSY whose mean rating is 3.86 or 8COG with 3.74 would be risky to interpret in a record with elevated Cl, TR, and/or ME. On the other hand, AMac (O-S rating = 2.63), OH (2.39), and 3DSA (2.10) can be interpreted with reasonable safety even in the faking bad record. In general, a scale with a mean item rating of less than 3.00 will be interpretable.

CHAPTER 4
THE ASSESSMENT
OF PSYCHOPATHOLOGY

There is still debate about whether the MMPI was originally intended to assess personality, but there is little doubt that a primary purpose was to assist in diagnosing psychopathology. The titles of the original clinical scales testified to this aim with abundant clarity. Hathaway and McKinley (1951, p. 6) stated flatly that "a high score on a scale has been found to predict positively the corresponding final clinical diagnosis or estimate in more than 60 per cent of new psychiatric admissions."

This optimistic prediction was never verified. In fact, it rapidly became clear that many psychiatric patients, especially those who were seriously disturbed, would be more likely to have two elevated clinical scales rather than a lone "spike." The concept of the 2-point code type was in place early on (Hathaway, 1947) and within a decade, was to become the orthodoxy. The official policy now was that assigning numbers to the scales was an attempt to escape from the misleading diagnostic connotations of the original scale labels. It was formally acknowledged that "it had become apparent with widespread testing that many people who scored high on the Sc scale were by no means clinically schizophrenic" (Welsh & Dahlstrom, 1956, p. 124). Coding now was advanced as "a positive approach to the clinical and research problems with the MMPI" (Welsh & Dahlstrom, 1956, p. 124).

The same "widespread testing" also demonstrated that code typology was not much more successful as a diagnostic tactic than the use of single scales. The next step was the development of rules based on all or most of the clinical scales such as those devised by Meehl and Dahlstrom (1960) and Goldberg (1965). These systems were designed not to make specific diagnoses but simply to distinguish among broad categories of diagnostic entities such as psychosis and neurosis.

A summary and extension of investigations of these diagnostic methods shows that they, too, have failed (Pancoast, Archer, & Gordon, 1988). The accuracy of diagnostic identification by several systems ranged from about one quarter to one third of cases examined, not very far from chance expectation and too weak to be of value to the practicing clinician.

THE MEASUREMENT OF SYMPTOMS

With the exception of the five-scale system created by Rosen (1962), special scales have not been devised for differential diagnosis and there has been no suggestion that they should be employed in this manner. Special scales are usually used to measure symptoms and occasionally, personality characteristics. Only a few of the large number of special scales that purport to assess symptoms have been evaluated either experimentally or clinically. In this chapter we will discuss some of those scales that have passed the test of clinical evaluation. An important consideration that needs to be discussed before proceeding is the distinction between *state* and *trait* measures.

MMPI Scales: State or Trait?

The distinction between an inventory item that measures an immediate, momentary state and one that taps a chronic, continuing characteristic like a trait is ordinarily evoked by instructions to the respondent. A classic example is the State-Trait Anxiety Inventory (Spielberger, Gorsuch, Lushene, Vagg, & Jacobs, 1983). Inventory items rarely have a self-contained message that permits a state or trait inference, like "right now, I feel . . .". Instead, instructions for completing the inventory will direct the respondent to answer "as you feel right now" (state) or "as you generally feel" (trait). This type of instruction is not part of the administration of the MMPI nor would it necessarily be desirable that it should be. The intent of administration of the inventory may be to assess state or trait; usually, it will make little difference. The evaluator will be equally interested in both kinds of assessments.

In the absence of specific instructions, almost all items appear as trait measures. Indeed, some of the MMPI items clearly suggest a trait by the inclusion in the item of terms like "at times" or "most of the time" or "frequently." Nevertheless, the respondent is free to make his/her own interpretation of whether the intent of the item is to measure trait or state. Fortunately, it appears to make little practical difference in the assessment of psychopathology. Generally, state and trait are highly correlated, usually in the vicinity of .60–.70. The correlation may be even higher when the respondents are mental patients.

Anxiety

No MMPI clinical scale is designed to measure anxiety although the role is often assigned to Scale 7. There are a number of special scales specifically created for this purpose. Unfortunately, clinical experience has not included all of them. The two best-known special scales intended to measure anxiety, Taylor's Manifest Anxiety Scale (MAS; Taylor, 1953) and Welsh's A Factor (Welsh, 1956) have not proven clinically useful. The primary reason in the case of the MAS is that it is heavily loaded with physical symptom items—13 of its 50. It has a marked tendency to elevate when the respondent is prone to somatize but does not have anxiety, worry, apprehension, and the like, as a primary symptom, except, perhaps, where their physical symptoms are concerned. The A Scale, in the light of today, appears to be a yea-saying measure of a tendency to psychological maladjustment that includes items that tap symptoms other than anxiety such as depression, guilt, hypersensitivity, and obsessive–compulsiveness. In fact, it appears that there are more depression items on the A Scale than items that measure anxiety directly.

Clinical usage suggests that the two most effective measures of anxiety among special scales are the Tryon, Stein, and Chu Tension Scale (TSC/T) and the Wiggins Phobias Scale (PHO). TSC/T measures nonspecific or free-floating anxiety as in a diagnosis of Generalized Anxiety Disorder. PHO is designed to tap the realm of sharply defined, specific fears. Unfortunately, it is by no means a simple matter to determine when a fear should be called a phobia (the reader is referred to the discussion on this point in Levitt, 1980b, pp. 6–8). Actually, it appears that no more than 15 of the 27 items in PHO qualify as phobias. But because the expected means on PHO are about 7 for men and about 10 for women, it would be most unusual to have a significant elevation on PHO without endorsement of a number of phobia items.

There is an overlap of 11 items between PHO and TSC/T. Of these 11 items, 4 are clearly not phobias, 3 are phobias and 4 others are questionable.

Item overlap, which amounts to 31% for TSC/T and 41% for PHO, unquestionably accounts partly for the correlation of .71 between the scales for both males and females. Obviously, we expect these two scales to cofluctuate, not only because of the item overlap but for sound theoretical reason. Most people who have high trait anxiety are also prone to specific fears. However, the employment of both scales is still useful because individuals who score high on one and do not elevate on the other are not rare. Some trait anxious individuals are worriers, people who have chronic minor-to-moderate anxiety but do not bind anxiety in highly specific fears. At the other end of the spectrum are individuals whose defenses do such an effective job of binding free-floating anxiety that it appears only as phobic.

Depression

Depression, the most commonly used term in the psychopathology lexicon, is a vastly complex phenomenon. Its complexities have been discussed elsewhere and we need go no further than to note that it is variably used to designate a temporary state which may be a symptom of some syndrome or diagnostic entity or a diagnosis in its own right (Levitt, Lubin, & Brooks, 1983). Some clinicians believe that not every depressed person is manifestly unhappy—the so-called masked depression. Some depressed patients benefit from chemotherapy, some do not. A few commit suicide but more than patients with other diagnoses.

Depression as a mood is clearly a state. Trait depression is more difficult to conceptualize. Logically, it must refer to a chronic, low grade condition or to recurrent episodes. The distinction between state and trait depression, like anxiety, does not seem important in interpreting MMPI records. The content of endorsed items has greater significance.

A problem with the MMPI Depression scale is that 13 of its items, more than 21%, deal with physical health. Physical symptoms abound among psychiatric patients, nonspecifically and most often do not distinguish between patients. Logically, a good depression measure should assess features other than the physical. Physical health can be evaluated with the appropriate Wiggins and Tryon, Stein, and Chu scales discussed in Chapter 3.

Physical symptom items are not included either in Wiggins' DEP, which has 33 items nor in TSC/D, which has 28. Thus, both of these are superior measures of the affective and cognitive aspects of depression.

DEP and TSC/D have a not surprising overlap of 14 items and an intercorrelation for both men and women of .94. Obviously, the two scales cofluctuate tightly with each other. In addition, they also have correlations ranging from .80 to .90 with Harris and Lingoes subscales 2SD (Subjective Depression) and 2MD (Mental Dullness). The correlations with 2PM range only from .39 to .43, which is a statistical illustration of the value of using depression scales that are not weighted with bodily symptom items.

Suicide Potential. One of the most significant assessments that is made by mental health professionals is the probability that a patient will commit suicide. The suicide rate among individuals diagnosed as depressives, schizophrenics, and alcoholics is significantly greater than the rate in the general population (Levitt, Lubin, & Brooks, 1983). A not infrequent rationale for hospitalization is that the individual appears to pose the threat of suicide. Thus, accurate prediction is extremely important and it is not surprising to find that a fair number of studies have been devoted to attempts to assess suicide potential using MMPI scales or items. Clopton (1979b) authored the most recent review of this literature.

Two inferences may be drawn from Clopton's review: (a) The clinical scales have been unsuccessful in predicting suicide potential; and (b) At least four suicide potential scales have independently developed from the MMPI item pool. None of these appears to be a successful measure of suicide potential.

Apparently, no one has tried to use already existing MMPI special scales to assess suicide potential. A popular hypothesis concerning the relationship between depression and suicide suggests that certain special scales may indeed be effective in predicting the suicide possibility.

This view holds that the depressed person contains within his/her symptomatology an essence that militates against self-destruction, namely, that the sufferer lacks the energy and drive to do away with him or herself. Improvement in the depressive symptoms may *increase* the suicide risk, a not uncommon clinical observation (for example, Pokorny, 1968; Klerman, 1982). As Pokorny (1968) pointed out, "the greatest risk of suicide is during the period of improvement; at this time the patient may regain sufficient drive or energy to take his life" (p. 71). It might be inferred that it is not only after improvement has taken place that risk heightens but at any time when the patient is badly disturbed but *not severely apathetic or anergic*.

The Psychomotor Retardation subscale of Scale 2 (2PR) contains the subset of depression items that tap apathy and anergy. The Subjective Depression subscale of Scale 2 (2SD) contains the depression items that deal with subjective feelings of unhappiness, guilt, worthlessness, and so on.[8] The correlation between 2PR and 2SD is only .38 for males, .56 for females, and .48 for the total sample. Some part of this relationship is surely due to an interscale overlap of eight items. Evidently, at least some individuals with high scores on 2SD are likely to have low scores on 2PR. This differential occurs among psychiatric patients as well as in normative groups.

Among depressed patients, those with the expected high scores on 2SD but with low scores on 2PR would logically be the suicide risks. Unfortunately, there has been no objective investigation of the possible predictive capacity of the 2PR-2SD combination. Clinical experience is scanty but there have been at least a few cases in which a score of T70 or higher on 2SD with a score of less than T60 on 2PR was associated with a suicide attempt. It is a worthwhile possibility to be checked out by the MMPI clinician.

Dysthymia/Trait Depression. Individuals who are depressed when the MMPI is administered will invariably treat the items in DEP and TSC/D as indicators of the current state. The depth of the depression is roughly related to the elevation of the scale. These measures, like 2SD, are composed entirely of obvious items. Interpretive accuracy is improved by evaluating these obvious-item scale scores against the subtle items of Scale 2, represented by Depression-Subtle (Wiener & Harmon, 1946).[9]

Every investigation has shown that the Depression-Obvious items and the Depression-Subtle items are either uncorrelated or have low negative correlations

---

[8]Notably, four of the 15 items in 2PR and 10 of the 32 items in 2SD—30% of the total number of items in these two scales—are included in the 52-item Suicide Threat scale developed by Farberow and Devries (1967).

[9]Depression-Subtle was the only one of the Wiener and Harmon subtle scales that was found to have any interpretive value.

(e.g., Wiener, 1956). The correlation between D-O and D-S was found by Wiener (1956) to be −.20 which is significant at the 1% level but the variance overlap—less than 5%—clearly indicates that these are independent measures for all practical purposes.

The absence of a meaningful correlation means that when D-O is elevated, D-S may be low, moderate, or high and vice versa. But these combinations are not random; on the contrary, they have interpretive significance.

The subtle items were included in the original MMPI pool because they were perceived clinically to be aspects of various syndromes despite having little or no face validity. What do the subtle items measure then?

Prolonged clinical experience strongly suggests that D-S is a measure of *trait depression*. Respondents who score in the vicinity of T60 on D-S are depression-prone individuals. They tend to experience depression as a state more often than most other depressed people. Usually, their scores on DEP and TSC/D are only moderately elevated, perhaps in the range T58–68. They are sometimes diagnosed as dysthymic.

Respondents who score above T70 on DEP and/or TSC/D are evidently seriously depressed, perhaps in the throes of a major depression. However, such individuals may or may not be trait depressed, and indeed will often have D-S scores below T55.

A singular characteristic of trait depressive individuals is that they seem to find living to be a trial even though they may have minimal feelings of being in a depressed mood, or of having guilt feelings or cognitive symptoms of depression. Matters do not necessarily go wrong for them; they just don't seem to go right. Such individuals seldom feel elated or attain a truly "up" mood and tend to be a bit cross and irritable more often than others.

Depression Without Guilt. A poor self-concept is a standard aspect of the depression syndrome. It is represented by MMPI items like "I certainly feel useless at times" and "I cannot do anything well." Assessment of self-concept independent of other aspects of depression is accomplished by means of the Wiggins Poor Morale scale (MOR) and the Indiana Self-Concept inventory (I-SC). Correlations between negativity on the self concept scales and depression scales like DEP and TSC/D are high. Correlations between DEP and MOR are regularly reported to be above .80 (e.g., Nichols, 1984) despite the fact that the two scales do not have any items in common.

While this kind of positive relationship is the general rule, it is not found invariably. There are several conditions in which a significant elevation on DEP and/or TSC/D will not be accompanied by the expected elevation on MOR or I-SC. This lack of correspondence is psychometrically possible because of the relative absence of item overlaps between the depression and the self-concept scales. For example, if the respondent endorsed every I-SC and MOR item that is in TSC/D, his/her self-concept scores would barely reach T50. A respondent's score on DEP could reach as high as T80 without a score on I-SC above T40.

Reactive depressions in individuals with no premorbid psychopathology are likely to have elevated depression scale scores without concomitant elevations of the self-concept scales. Individuals with chronic pain syndromes or chronic or progressive or life-threatening illnesses or disabilities also manifest this pattern. This is clearly one of the many instances of the utility of special scales in contrast to the isolated use of the conventional MMPI clinical scale.

The Measurement of Psychoticism

Beyond the structural defects of MMPI clinical scales noted in Chapter 1, the identification of psychoticism by means of a verbal inventory is always risky and must be tentative. Response sets, poor reading ability, and the opportunity for misunderstandings and idiosyncratic interpretation of items accumulate to plague the clinician in the identification of thought disorders and other severe psychopathology.

The MMPI clinical scales have been no more successful in the diagnosis of psychoticism than might be expected. The F Scale, long heralded as a psychotic measure in its own right, frequently elevates when the respondent is psychotic—and often elevates when the respondent is not. Any respondent with a significant elevation on Scale 8, either alone as a spike or in conjunction with Scales 6 and 7, is commonly considered to be schizophrenic. However, there is no doubt whatsoever that a substantial number of people who show elevations on Scale 8 are not psychotic.

There are several other methods of combining clinical scale scores in order to attempt to measure psychoticism, such as Peterson's (1954) six diagnostic signs and Goldberg's (1965) index. None of these attempts has proven sufficiently successful to warrant their common use in clinical facilities.

Obviously, special scales are not immune to the problems of the verbal instrument but at least they have the potential to avoid some of the structural defects of the clinical scales. There are six special scales that have potential utility in diagnosing thought disorder.

Indiana Severe Reality Distortion Scale (I-RD)

I-RD is a face valid instrument that is composed simply of the 18 hallucinations and delusions that are in the MMPI item pool. To be sure, these may be misunderstood; indeed the means of between 1 and 2 for both males and females on this scale in themselves suggest misunderstandings. However, a raw score of 5 for women or 6 for men (that is, T70) is unlikely to be due to item misinterpretations and appears to be pathognomic of a psychotic process.

The Indiana Dissociative Symptoms Scale (I-DS)

I-DS is another face valid scale which is composed of the eight items in the MMPI pool that describe dissociative symptoms such as "I have had periods in which I carried on activities without knowing later what I had been doing," or

"I often feel as if things are not real." I-DS contains three I-RD items. This necessitates caution since T70 for males on I-DS is only 3 and for females, 4. Thus, in order to be certain that I-DS is contributing to the symptomatology beyond the score obtained on I-RD, the score on I-DS would have to exceed T70.

While symptoms in I-DS are usually classified as dissociative, they are not infrequently found in psychotic persons. Consider, for example, items such as "My soul sometimes leaves my body," and "I have had some very unusual religious experiences."

Wiggins' Psychoticism Scale (PSY)

PSY numbers among its 48 items all 18 in I-RD, and eight items that form the Harris and Lingoes Bizarre Sensory Experiences subscale of Scale 8 (8BSE). These 26 items, a bit more than half of the complement in PSY, may be considered to be legitimate measures of psychoticism. However, PSY also contains nine items that appear either in 4SOA or 8SOA, or in both. Among sociopathic, disillusioned, or otherwise alienated persons, a high score on 4SOA or 8SOA can cause PSY to elevate spuriously. This is especially true because the overlap of PSY items on either alienation scale is almost equal to a standard deviation unit of PSY. Thus, in assessing the significance of PSY, one must examine the two alienation scales. If they are elevated, then there is a good probability that a high score on PSY does not indicate the presence of psychoticism. On the other hand, if 4SOA and 8SOA are within the normal range, then an elevation on PSY could be pathognomic of a psychotic process.

Paranoia. TSC/S assesses distrustfulness across a broad range of psychological adjustments. It measures suspiciousness as a common trait variable in the general population. High scorers are likely to be suspicious, cynical, and opportunistic with status ranging from normal to sociopathic. They are not likely to be delusional or paranoid in the classical sense. Consider, for example, the diagnostic difference between "Someone has it in for me," which is like the sociopathic externalization of blame and the "Someone is trying to poison me" of the paranoid schizophrenic.

Several special scales are sensitive to paranoid ideation in the respondent, for example, PSY, 6PI, and 8COG. None of these is sufficiently specific. Perhaps one-third of the 17 items of 6PI tap paranoia directly, fewer on PSY and 8COG. A diagnosis involving paranoid ideation is made with reasonable confidence based on a high score on the Extreme Suspiciousness Scale (S+; Endicott, Jortner, & Abramoff, 1969). About half of the 18 items on S+ are clearly paranoid delusions. The remaining items express the hypersensitivity and hypercaution that are likely to underlie paranoid tendencies. High scorers on S+ are paranoid persons at some level. Not all are psychotic; some will be diagnosed as paranoid personality disorders (see discussion in Chapter 5).

The Measurement of Antisocial Tendency

The behaviors of the antisocial personality disorder as they are described in DSM-III-R (APA, 1987) are essentially those of a criminal and/or vagrant: lying, cheating, pursuing an illegal occupation, failing to plan ahead, wandering without good purpose from place to place, unable to sustain any socially productive or responsible behavior, and generally not following social norms. This pattern is seen in an estimated 3% of the adult population, mostly males, according to DSM-III-R.

There are others who manifest tendencies like the antisocial personality but not necessarily to a psychopathological extreme. Many are not criminals or vagrants and do not warrant a diagnosis of antisocial personality disorder. Even the term *antisocial* appears somewhat amiss when applied to such individuals. The original DSM term *sociopathic* (APA, 1952) seems to describe them more clearly.

These individuals have personality structures that resemble the antisocial personality disorder. They are apt to feel misunderstood and put upon, to externalize blame, to be rebellious, cynical, and suspicious of the motivations of others. Most have never been able to build an effective social support system and usually feel isolated, alone, and perhaps different. Guilt is rarely a prominent feature but hostility and/or depression may be manifested. Yet, a large number of individuals with sociopathic tendencies manage to function without intervention and without attracting the attention of authorities of any kind.

Items tapping sociopathic tendencies will be found on Scales 4 and 6 of the MMPI but typically, indistinguishable in a melange of items measuring other characteristics. Certainly, sociopathically inclined persons may elevate on Scale 4 but as we saw in Chapter 1, high scores on this scale may also be obtained by individuals without particular tendency toward sociopathy.

There are 10 special scales that are involved in the identification of the respondent with sociopathic inclinations. Four are Harris and Lingoes subscales: 4AC, 4SOA, 8SOA, and 9AMO; two are in the Wiggins group: AUT and HOS; two are Tryon, Stein, and Chu scales: TSC/R and TSC/S. The complement is completed by the Cook and Medley (1954) Ho scale and Eichman's (1961) Cynicism Scale (E/Cy).

Alienation.   The cornerstone scales in this group are 4SOA and 8SOA which generally cofluctuate despite the fact that they have only four items—approximately 20% of each scale—in common. High scorers on these scales typically feel isolated and lack an effective support system. They also feel generally misunderstood and tend to externalize blame for their problems. Individuals who score above T70 on either scale have a strong sense of being estranged from society and feel discriminated against as well as misunderstood.

These individuals also often score high on the two scales that assess family difficulties: the Harris and Lingoes Familial Discord subscale (4FD) and Wiggins'

Family Problems Scale (FAM). Incidentally, the family difficulties scales cofluctuate markedly due to an overlap of eight items which amounts to 50% of the items in FAM and more than 70% of the ones in 4FD.

Suspiciousness.   TSC/S measures suspiciousness as a nonpsychotic tendency. Individuals who score in the range T55–T65 on TSC/S tend to be hypercautious and controlled in their interpersonal dealings. Those who score above T65 must be considered to be suspicious people who often question the motives and intentions of others and tend to be doubtful about the purposes of rules and the dicta of authority figures.

A diagnosis of antisocial personality disorder can be made only against the backdrop of behavioral information. Certain types of criminals are highly likely to produce a rash of elevations of T65 and T70 on the 10 sociopathic tendency scales. However, every respondent with this pattern of scales is not necessarily a criminal.

Cynicism.   Frequent accompaniments of alienation are cynicism and suspicion. E/Cy is a relatively pure measure of cynicism, whereas Ho, as indicated in an earlier discussion, taps an amalgam of cynicism and hostility. The overlap between the two scales amounts to 14% for Ho and 27% for E/Cy.

Harris and Lingoes 9AMO tends to elevate with all of the scales mentioned so far, especially the measures of cynicism. Individuals scoring high on 9AMO tend to perceive others as behaving dishonestly, selfishly, and opportunistically and therefore feel justified in behaving similarly. It reflects a kind of a jungle philosophy in which one either takes advantage of others or is taken advantage of by others.

Anger.   The best measure of experienced hostility is Wiggins' HOS. Individuals who elevate on this scale are aware of their hostility although they may not be aware that it is manifested as often as it actually is. The Tryon, Stein, and Chu Resentment Scale (TSC/R) is also a measure of hostility but of a somewhat different tenor. The anger of people who score high on TSC/R has a pettish, irritable quality, much like an adolescent who reacts negatively to the impression that he/she is being put upon, manipulated, and overpowered by his/her parents. Indeed, adolescents are more likely to elevate on TSC/R than are adults.

Authority Conflict.   The two measures of authority conflict—AUT and 4AC—have only three items in common and appear to tap somewhat different aspects of this phenomenon. The correlation between the two scales is only .38 for females and .41 for males and indeed, clinically one sees a substantial number of instances in which 4AC is significantly elevated and AUT is not. Such individuals are unaware of their rebellious inclinations, unlike high scorers on AUT who seem to be aware. Significantly, the correlation between AUT and HOS is .66 for females and .64 for males while the correlation between 4AC and HOS is only .26 and .23.

Special Problems

Two conditions that the psychologist is often called upon to diagnose are substance abuse and sexual difficulties. The supply of special scales fortunately contains several scales that have outstanding clinical track records in these areas.

Substance Abuse: The MacAndrew Alcoholism Scale (AMac). A number of scales have been developed from MMPI items to identify alcoholics. A 49-item scale developed by MacAndrew (1965) has rightly received the most attention.[10] Almost without exception, field tests have upheld the capacity of the AMac to distinguish male alcoholics from various nonalcoholic samples (Apfeldorf & Hunley, 1975; Rhodes, 1969; Rich & Davis, 1969; Uecker, 1970; Vega, 1971; Whisler & Cantor, 1966). Clinical experience supported by research findings indicates that AMac also identifies substance abusers in general (Burke & Marcus, 1977; Kranitz, 1972; Lachar, Berman, Grisell, & Schoof, 1976) as well as substance abusers in an inactive stage either because abuse has not yet been initiated (Hoffmann, Loper, & Kammeier, 1974; Huber & Danahy, 1975) or because it is no longer a problem.

Views on the appropriate cutting score for AMac vary. A raw score of 24 for males is in common use, based on MacAndrew's (1965) original work supported by later independent investigations (e.g., Burke & Marcus, 1977). Lachar et al. (1976) reported that a cut-off of 23 was more efficient. Svanum, Levitt, and McAdoo (1982) recommended 25 as the cutting score based on regression analyses.

Cut-off points are always slippery matters, especially when "alcoholic–drug addict" lies on one side and "not alcoholic or drug addict" on the other. Caution must be a paramount consideration.

Means of approximately 23 have been reported for inpatient males without substance problems in several studies (e.g., Burke & Marcus, 1977; Lachar et al., 1976). Svanum et al. (1982) reported a mean of 21.5 with an SD of 5.1. The mean AMac score for males in the Indiana normative sample is 25.08 with an SD of 4.89. Gottesman, Hanson, Kroeker, and Briggs (1987) reported a mean of 23 for normal 18-year-old males. Potential control guidelines thus range from around 22 to 25.

Mean scores for alcoholics have been reported as 27 (Burke & Marcus, 1977), 28 (Lachar et al., 1976) and 30 (Svanum et al., 1982). Comparing these means with the data for possible control samples, it is plain that a cutting score of 23 or 24 will identify most of the alcoholics but with a considerable volume of false positives.

In the Burke and Marcus sample of nonsubstance abuse inpatients who were also not schizophrenic, a score of 28.2 would be T60. T60 in the Lachar et al. control samples would be 28.7 for alcoholics, 28.4 for heroin addicts, and 26.2

---

[10] The scale originally contained 51 items including the two that deal directly with alcohol use. Conventionally, these two items are not included in AMac.

for polydrug users. In the Svanum et al. study, 26.57 would correspond to T60 in the control sample. T60 in the Indiana sample would be a score of 29.97; it would be 27 in the Gottesman et al. sample.

There is no mathematical way to accumulate all these data so as to arrive at an absolute measure of central tendency. From inspection, it would appear that a score of 28 is a reasonable cut-off point for males. It should be pointed out, however, that cases of alcoholics with scores as low as 25 are not uncommon in clinical practice (see, for example, the case in Table 3.6).

The Svanum et al. (1982) investigation is one of the rare ones that has furnished data on female alcoholics. They reported a mean of 26.72 for alcoholics and 19.45 for a control group of inpatient nonalcoholics with a recommended cutting score of 23. The AMac mean for females in the Indiana sample is 23.32, SD = 4.58. The Gottesman et al. (1987) 18-year-old females had a mean AMac score of 20 with 24 as T60.

Evidently, there is some agreement that females in general score lower on AMac than males. A cut-off of 25 for females would appear reasonable but again, it must be noted that alcoholic females with scores of 23 and 24 are encountered in clinical practice.

Sexual Problems: The Pedophilia Scale (Pe) and the Indiana Sex Problems Scales. The Pe Scale was developed by contrasting records of 120 male pedophiles incarcerated in a California prison with 160 prisoners who had not been convicted of a sexual crime (Toobert, Bartelme, & Jones, 1959). The consequent comparison yielded 24 items that differentiated the two groups at the 5% level or beyond. These items form the Pe Scale.

Toobert et al. (1959) then proceeded to cross-validate the scale on a sample of 38 pedophiles who were not included in the original development of the scale and a group of 50 general prisoners which had also not been previously tested. A sample of 65 psychiatric patients in an Army hospital was also included in the cross-validation.

In both the original and the cross-validation study, the pedophiles scored higher on Pe than any of the other groups. The authors note that a cutting score of 8 on Pe identified approximately 75% of the pedophiles with false positives in the other groups ranging from 20 to 42%.

The Indiana normative data suggest that the cut-off is too low. The mean Pe in the Indiana sample was 6.92 with an SD of 2.46. A raw score of 10 is equivalent to T63, a status of suspicion but not certainty. T71, which would appear to be highly diagnostic, is attained by a raw score of 12.

In clinical practice, Pe has proven to be an outstandingly successful measuring instrument. Its ability to identify is not restricted to pedophiles. High scorers may also be exhibitionists or voyeurs. This is not surprising if one considers that the control groups in the developmental studies did not include paraphiliacs other than pedophiles. Thus, the Pe Scale appears to be identifying common characteristics of several groups of paraphiliacs. Examination of the scale suggests that the tendencies that are tapped by the scale are in accordance with the backward personalities of pedophiles, exhibitionists, and voyeurs as they have been unravelled in clinical examination (see for example, Gebhard, Gagnon, Pomeroy, & Christenson, 1965).

Although the Indiana Sex Problems Scale has been discussed in a previous chapter, it is presented again in its proper context. As previously noted, high scorers on I-SP are likely to have a sexual problem, often a dysfunction such as impotence, anorgasmia, sexual aversiveness, or sexual preoccupation. These different conditions are not distinguished by the scale score per se but can often be determined when I-SP is elevated from responses to individual items. For example, "Sexual things disgust me" suggests aversiveness or anorgasmia and "There is something wrong with my sexual organs" may indicate a male dysfunction.

CONFLICT

Some scales are highly positively correlated because of heavy overlap of items. An outstanding example is FAM and 4FD which have eight items in common—50% of the items in FAM and more than 70% of 4FD. The correlation of .80 is hardly unexpected. Other scale pairs cofluctuate either positively or negatively due to the nature of the variables involved rather than to item overlap. One would expect, for example, E/Cy and 9AMO to be positively related despite no item overlap and they are (.41). On the other side of the ledger, we should find that I-De and I-Do are negatively related and they are (−.36) with only one common item, keyed differently on the two scales.

In the individual record, scale pairs that would be expected to be either positively or negatively correlated may actually be unrelated. But scale pairs are seldom related in the direction opposite to expectation in the individual record. When this occurs, we find that the respondent has a serious conflict in the area represented by the scale pair.

Values

The usual indicators of the moral–virtuous patterns are elevations of 3NA, 6N, and, sometimes, the L Scale (see Chapter 5). The negatively related scale, 9AMO, would be expected to be below the normal range.

When 9AMO is also elevated, the pattern is an indication of an intense conflict in the area of moral values. The respondent is desperately seeking to maintain his/her perception of him/herself as a righteous person but at the same time is beset by doubts that morality is warranted in an immoral society. If the respondent is a woman and I-SP is also elevated, the conflict may involve a press to act out sexually. This is especially likely to be the case if the respondent is married although the conflict is also found in single women.

Social Anxiety and Social Stimulation

Individuals who score high on 9PMA have a high optimal stimulation level, a greater than average need for involving themselves in situations that are stimulating, pleasurably exciting. A few of us drive cars very fast or climb mountains. But for most people, stimulation is social; it is provided by interrelationships, by associating with others. The high 9PMA person who has no difficulty socializing is able to satisfy his/her need for stimulation. The respondent who elevates on 9PMA but also is high on SOC and/or TSC/I and is a low scorer on 3DSA, 4SI, and/or 9IMP, has an emotionally upsetting problem. These individuals are apt to be socially maladroit and anxious, are shy, embarrass easily, are awkward in social situations, and do not make friends easily. Thus, they have difficulty in gratifying the high optimum stimulation level. This is more likely to be true when the respondent is an adult, less likely in the case of an adolescent for whom the conflict may very well become de-emphasized by further emotional development.

Hostility Control

The individual who characteristically overcontrols hostility by denial and repression is likely to elevate on OH. Typically, this person will have a low score on hostility scales, especially HOS and AUT. The individual who characteristically denies hostility perceives himself/herself as a placid individual not given to anger. In some people, the denial mechanism is faulty even though the need to overcontrol is strong. Such individuals are not only high scorers on OH but also on scales like HOS. The conflict between the need to control hostility and the need to express it is likely to be painful and is apt to be reflected in elevations on symptom scales.

Dependency–Suspicion

Dependent people rely on others to make decisions, to establish goals, and generally to assume responsibility for their lives. To be successfully dependent (bear with the contradiction in terms), one must be naive and trusting. A chronically cynical, suspicious person obviously has difficulty in establishing relationships and thus cannot fulfill dependency needs. The conflict of needs is usually experienced in late adolescence or early adulthood and brings symptoms with it.

A typical instance is the 19-year-old female college student whose T-scores on I-De and I-Do were 59 and 38 respectively—a characteristic pair of scores for the dependent person. Unfortunately, she also had scores of T59 on TSC/S, T66 on S+, and T66 on E/Cy. She came into outpatient psychotherapy with depression as presenting complaint: DEP = T75; TSC/D = T79; also I-SC = T78, and MOR = T74. At the end of a year—40 visits—her depression scores were essentially unchanged, a tribute to the suspiciousness that made it impossible for her to participate in a therapeutic alliance.

PROGNOSIS

The Control Scale (Cn)

Some seriously emotionally disturbed individuals urgently require hospitalization. Others, whose symptoms appear to be serious, maintain themselves in the community, at least marginally. How to tell one from the other, to determine who needs (expensive) hospitalization and who does not, is a perennial clinical problem.

An MMPI approach to this problem was attempted by Cuadra (1956). Cuadra decided on a contrasting group approach, simple in conception, but tedious to carry out as carefully as Cuadra did. The first step was to select 30 young, reasonably well-educated psychiatric patients who had voluntarily sought treatment and were tested within 15 days of admission. These "criterion abnormals" were then matched with a group of "criterion normals," which was Cuadra's way of describing a group that was equally as disturbed but for whom hospitalization had not been recommended. The two groups were essentially similar in age and education and were almost identical in scores on MMPI clinical and validity scales. Cuadra had to sift through 4,000 records in order to obtain his criterion normals!

Cuadra's Control Scale (Cn) consists of 32 items which had discriminated the two criterion groups best for both sexes plus an additional 18 items which did not differentiate the criterion groups quite as effectively but did discriminate them in the same direction for both sexes. There was little overlap in the total scale scores between Cuadra's criterion groups. The range of scores for the "normal" was 27–45; for the "abnormals" 9–33. Only four scores in the normal group were below 30; only one of the abnormals was above 30.

Forty-four of the 50 items on Cn are found on one or another of the clinical scales or the F Scale. One of the psychometric advantages of Cn is that of these 40 items, 19 are keyed in the direction opposite to the conventional scoring. Thus, an individual does not automatically elevate on Cn simply by endorsing psychopathological items.

Inspection of the scale suggests that high scorers on the scale will have a greater tendency to admit to relatively minor behavioral shortcomings and to be less religious than low scorers.

The scale can be used in accordance with its original intention, that is, low scorers with serious psychopathology should be hospitalized; high scorers (above T65) are better able to subsist on an outpatient basis. However, a high score does not necessarily rule out a "faking bad" response posture, as Cuadra originally suggested, probably because most of the items in the scale are not endorsed in the deviant direction by individuals who are faking bad.

Work Attitude Scale

A significant aspect of emotional illness, one that is sometimes neglected by diagnosticians, is the patient's subjective feeling of incapacity. Certainly there are multiple factors involved in a person's belief that he/she has lost the ability to work productively in whatever setting. Surely one of the most important is the subjective feeling that symptomatology is so overpowering that cognitive and intellectual capacities are stifled and motivation is undermined.

The Work Attitude Scale (WA; Tydlaska & Mengel, 1953) measures this feeling with reasonable accuracy. The scale was originally developed by contrasting groups of industrial employees who had received regular merit ratings of "satisfactory" over a 2-year period with a group of Air Force personnel, most of whom had gone AWOL or were disciplinary problems.

Fifty-eight items were selected by judges (not otherwise described) on the basis of estimated potential for distinguishing between the two groups. Items that dealt with sociopathic behavior such as alcohol abuse and difficulties with authorities were eliminated on the grounds that although they might very well discriminate the two groups, they would not be helpful for the purposes of the proposed scale.

MMPIs of the two groups were now examined and it was found that 37 of the 58 selected items discriminated at the 1% level. These became the Work Attitude Scale (WA). The mean WA score for the Air Force personnel was 16.4, for the industrial employees, 7.0. All but one of the former had scores above 10 while nearly 80% of the latter had scores below 10.

The scale was subsequently cross-validated on college student samples (Tesseneer & Tydlaska, 1956). Faculty members at a small state college selected 26 male students with whom they were personally familiar and whom they identified "as outstanding examples of good work attitudes." An equal number of students was selected as representing "poor work attitudes" by the faculty. The mean ages and IQs were essentially similar. The poor work attitude students were found to have a mean WA of 13.1 compared to 7.3 for the good work attitude students. The former were also found to have more psychopathology in general as measured by the clinical scales of the MMPI but, of course, this does impeach the validity of WA. It simply suggests that one effective interference with academic achievement is emotional upset.

Examination of the 37 items of WA indicates that a plurality—10—are found on DEP and TSC/D. Somewhat smaller groups are found in 2MD and 8CON. In fact, these are exactly the components that would be anticipated for this scale: dysphoric affect, interference with cognitive processes, and lack of motivation.

Patients who score in the range T60–69 on WA are complaining that their daily life functioning is impaired to some degree but not enough to require hospitalization. Scores of T70 and above indicate that emotional disturbance is sufficiently intense so that the patient feels that he/she cannot function productively. Hospitalization or medication may be requisite, depending on the level of Cn.

Alienation and Suspicion

Patients who score high on TSC/S and/or S+, especially T70 or above, do not make "good" patients. They doubt the benevolent intentions of the psychotherapist and are unlikely to develop sufficient trust and confidence to effectuate a productive course of therapy. The prognosis is even poorer when there are accompanying elevations on the alienation scales 4SOA, 8SOA, and Ho, not unusual cofluctuations. Such individuals are cynical, demanding, and externalize blame. They resist therapeutic efforts designed to move them to assume responsibility for their own behavior. Patients with high scores on any two of these five scales have a poor prognosis with any talking therapy.

Avoidant Tendency

The patient who scores low on 3DSA, 4SI, and 9IMP and high on SOC and TSC/I will have difficulty relating to a therapist in a productive fashion. Typically, such patients have trouble communicating verbally, especially the expression of feelings. The process of therapy is slow and a therapist requires unusual patience. Patients with low scores on at least one of the social comfort scales and a high score on at least one of the social introversion scales have a guarded prognosis with talking therapies.

CHAPTER 5
THE MEASUREMENT OF ADJUSTMENT AND PERSONALITY

It is possible that the creators of the MMPI regarded it as an all-purpose instrument that would assess personality as well as diagnose emotional disorder. The occurrence of the word "personality" itself in the title is suggestive. Perhaps the ambition was limited, a thought that might follow from the expression of purpose "to assay those traits that are commonly characteristic of disabling psychological abnormality" (Hathaway & McKinley, 1951, p. 5). Mental health professionals have employed the MMPI in all ways: as a diagnostic instrument, as a measure of emotional adjustment, and as a technique for personality assessment. No matter how it is used, the major shortcoming of the MMPI clinical scales intrudes on the accuracy and utility of results. The multidimensionality of the clinical scales makes diagnosis difficult; it interferes to even a greater degree with assessment of personality and adjustment. The Harris and Lingoes scales illustrate the extent to which logical fractionation of the clinical scales improves evaluation.

High-point code typologies are of less value in personality assessment than in diagnostic evaluation, no matter what stance one assumes with respect to interpretation. Greene (1980) remarked that studies of MMPI high points have typically been restricted to scales that were T70 or above. Then what could one say about the respondent whose profile was entirely below T60?

Graham (1977) at one time adopted a radical position that overlooked the weakness of code typology. He contended that *absolute elevations* of the scales in a two-point code are irrelevant. "A careful examination of the existing literature," claimed Graham, "suggests that in most cases the same basic extra-test behavioral correlates emerge for two-point codes irrespective of the order of the two scales and their absolute and relative elevations" (Graham, 1977, p. 64).

This concept of the two-point pair is indefensible. Many psychologists might agree with Graham that 48/84 persons "are seen by others as odd, peculiar, and queer . . . their behavior is erratic and unpredictable . . . prostitution, promiscuity, and sexual deviation are fairly common among 48/84 individuals" (Graham, 1977, p. 74; 1987, pp. 108–109). Most of those psychologists would have reference to a profile in which Scales 4 and 8 were T70 or above. One can hardly imagine a clinician who would render Graham's interpretation when the high-point pair was T60 or below. In fact, Graham has since shifted positions and currently agrees that "the descriptors presented for a particular code type are more likely to fit a subject with that code type if the two scales in the code type are elevated above T = 70" (Graham, 1987, p. 98).

High-point code typologies may have some utility when the high points are very high simply because more of the items in each scale have evoked the deviant response. Much of the elaborate library of statements that follows face validly from the content of scale items is more likely to be applicable to the respondent. The lower the scale elevations, the less probable it becomes that any set of personality and symptom descriptors will be applicable to the individual respondent.

The greater versatility and homogeneity of MMPI special scales improves personality assessment just as it does for diagnostic capacity. This chapter discusses the evaluation of some personality traits using special scales. Before that undertaking, it is obligatory to acknowledge that special scales cannot evaluate adjustment except in the restricted sense of asymptomatology. Psychologists who have some familiarity with special scales may believe otherwise. It is for this reason that the following discussion is included in this book.

THE MEASUREMENT OF PSYCHOLOGICAL ADJUSTMENT: A FAILURE OF THE MMPI ITEM POOL

The concept of *ego strength*, or *ego resources*, or *ego control* (perhaps the best term since it indicates not only strength but implies that the ego dominates the less corticate id and superego) has been an important construct in psychological theory since the early days of Freud. The underlying notion is that the ego, the reality oriented part of the personality, successfully controls the impulses emanating from the id and the superego whose capacities to perceive reality are limited, thus a definition in effect of mental and emotional health. Few question the value of the construct in theory. So it is not surprising that one of the first special scales emerging from the MMPI pool was an Ego-Strength Scale (Es; Barron, 1953).

Barron's Es consists of 68 items that differentiated 17 outpatients at a Veterans' Administration clinic who improved with a regimen of psychotherapy from 16 patients who did not improve. Improvement ratings were made by two expert judges on the basis of available documents. From the vantage point of 25 years later, Barron's methodology appears somewhat primitive. Sophisticated researchers now view psychotherapy outcome as a dimension or a process, not a dichotomy. But there is a more compelling reason to anticipate that any effort to measure strength of ego in a meaningful way using MMPI items is doomed to failure.

There are two ways to view the ego. In one conception, the individual who is high in ego power has a superior psychological adjustment, perhaps approaching an ideal such as that of Maslow's self-actualizing person (Lowry, 1973; Maslow, 1968). Contemporary constructs that would be synonymous with such a level of ego are *hardiness* (Kobasa, 1979, 1982) and *high-level wellness* (Ardell, 1977; Greenberg, 1985). High-level wellness and hardiness had no place in Freudian theory. Freud believed that ego-strength enables the individual to avoid symptoms; happiness was merely the escape from pain. Hardiness has surplus meaning beyond being asymptomatic. A measure of ego-strength that was more than simply the ability to avoid symptoms could have multiple important uses. It would be an effective measure of therapy progress and outcome and a prime tool for the selection of applicants for a wide variety of professions and occupations that require maturity. Unfortunately, it is literally impossible to construct such a subinventory from the MMPI pool.

A majority of the items in the MMPI pool are symptom statements. The respondent denies the presence of symptoms by responding "false" to the item, for example:

Most of the time I wish I were dead.
I am afraid when I look down from a high place.

A smaller set of items are keyed so that a "true" response indicates denial of a symptom, for example:

I usually feel that life is worthwhile.
I do not have a great fear of snakes.

Some items allege an equivalence of health or lack of symptoms with a norm, that is, the respondent indicates that he/she is normal, for example:

I am in just as good physical health as most of my friends.
I believe I am no more nervous than most others.

A few items affirm that the respondent's current state has not suffered across time, for example:

I am about as able to work as I ever was.
My eyesight is as good as it has been for years.

Basically, these types of items, which make up the bulk of the MMPI pool, either endorse or deny symptoms, nothing more. They cannot possibly be perceived as measuring a state that is reflected in a concept like hardiness. There are no more than a half-dozen MMPI items that could, in the broadest definition, be viewed as measuring a supernormality:

I have a good appetite.
I wake up fresh and rested most mornings.
My daily life is full of things that keep me interested.
I enjoy many different kinds of play and recreation.
I am entirely self-confident.
It is great to be living in these times when so much is going on.

The appetite item is the only one of the six that is included in Es although it would hardly seem to matter since all six would constitute less than 10% of the items in Es.

Nevertheless, Es has been the most widely used special scale by clinicians (Moreland & Dahlstrom, 1983) and is one of the rare special scales that has been the subject of a fair amount of experimental scrutiny. In view of the stuff of which Es is made, it should come as no surprise that the research hardly justifies its clinical use. It is surprising that Es has received so much research attention while Block's ego-control and ego-resiliency scales (Block, 1965), also composed of MMPI items, have been largely neglected. The methodology of development of the Block scales is superior to that of Es although they are no more likely to be successful construct measures.

Studies suggesting evidence for the validity of Es are of two types: (a) emotionally disturbed persons are shown to score lower than normal people (Taft, 1957; Quay, 1955; Kleinmuntz, 1960) although not invariably (Winter & Stortroen, 1963); (b) Es distinguishes between criterion groups according to hypothesis but so do other MMPI scales or scales composed of MMPI items (e.g., King-Ellison Good, 1957; Grosz & Levitt, 1959; Van Evra & Rosenburg, 1963; Snow & Held, 1973).

Such findings are unconvincing. Any set of 68 randomly selected MMPI items would have a high probability of distinguishing between patients and normals. Significantly, Es has demonstrated poor capacity to discriminate among patients with various diagnoses associated with degrees of severity (e.g., Tamkin & Klett, 1957; Tamkin, 1957; Sinnett, 1962; Hawkinson, 1961; Rosen, 1963; Shipman, 1965). The fact that other MMPI scales also discriminate suggests that discrimination is a function of nonspecific item content; it occurs simply because the MMPI as an instrument measures psychopathology or absence of psychopathology.

In addition to the studies already cited, evidence for lack of validity for Es is generally more convincing. Included are several unsuccessful attempts to find positive relationships between Es and Rorschach measures of ego-strength (e.g., Tamkin, 1957; Levine & Cohen, 1962; Adams & Cooper, 1962; Adams, Cooper, & Carrera, 1963; Herron, Guido, & Kantor, 1965; Barger & Sechrest, 1961). Even more damaging are several investigations in which Es was unsuccessful in predicting treatment outcome (e.g., Crumpton, Cantor, & Batiste, 1960; Levine & Cohen, 1962; Hawkinson, 1961). Crumpton et al. (1960) also found that while a student sample had a higher mean Es score than a patient sample, the overlap in distributions was so great that the most predictive cut-off score—which identified 97% of the students—did no better than chance at identifying patients. These researchers add that their findings "suggest strongly that the Barron ego strength scale is misnamed. Inspection of the content reveals that the scale takes a negative approach to the measurement of ego strength, i.e., the absence of indications of ego weakness is interpreted as ego strength ... 'ego weakness' would be a better term of what the scale is measuring than the term 'ego strength' ... the construct of ego strength should imply more than merely the absence of specific weaknesses" (Crumpton et al., 1960, p. 290).

Greene (1991) declined to provide interpretations of Es scores because "the contradictory nature of the research on the Es scale makes it inappropriate" (p. 187). Archer (1987) warned that "the use of the Es scale is clearly controversial for both adults and adolescent populations, and MMPI interpreters who employ this measure should be aware that predictions from the Es scale are often likely to be misleading in term of treatment prognosis" (p. 126).

In view of the nature of the MMPI item pool, the conclusions of Crumpton et al., Archer's warning, and Greene's caution were inevitable. The MMPI does not contain a subset of items that can assess psychological adjustment except in the limited sense that the term is synonymous with an absence of symptoms.

Despite the failure to measure psychological adjustment, special scales do a decent job of assessing *social* adjustment and certain personality characteristics and patterns.

THE MEASUREMENT OF SOCIAL ADJUSTMENT

There is no effective, single measure of social adjustment–maladjustment among the MMPI clinical scales although Scale 0 is often regarded as such an index. The study by deMendonca et al. (1984) shows that conventional interpretations of Scale 0 use such terms as *aloof, reserved, retiring, shy*, and *withdrawn* for high scorers on this scale and *sociable, friendly*, and *outgoing* for low scorers.

But terms like *inhibited* and *uninhibited, self-confident, friendly, sociable,* and *withdrawn* have also been used as descriptors of high and low scorers on clinical scales other than Scale 0.

A content analysis of Scale 0 by Serkownek (Schuerger et al., 1987) suggests that it is as multifaceted as other MMPI clinical scales. Even though the dimension of social adjustment–maladjustment is very broad, some of the Serkownek subscales are not located on the dimension. This finding is consonant with some of the early studies cited in Dahlstrom, Welsh, and Dahlstrom (1972) which reported that some of the terms also used to characterize high scorers on Scale 0 were modest, sensitive, natural, serious, kind, affectionate, soft-hearted, sentimental, stereotyped, lacking originality, permissive, and generally insecure.

There are some eight special scales that have bearing on the social adjustment–maladjustment continuum. Most of these scales show item overlap and moderate to high intercorrelations.

Three Harris and Lingoes scales measure social poise and comfort; low scorers on 3DSA, 4SI, and 9IMP tend to be socially anxious and maladroit. Since there are only 26 items represented in these three scales, one must anticipate at least two elevated above T60 before a statement can be made about social anxiety. 4SI is likely to be the most reliable of the three since it has the most items.

Two other scales measure schizoid tendency: Wiggins' SOC and the Tryon, Stein, and Chu Social Introversion Scale (TSC/I). Since the item overlap amounts to more than 50% for each scale, it is expected that they will cofluctuate markedly. But as it is so often the case in the use of special scales in a pattern, it is always more convincing and thus more diagnostically warranted when more than one scale assessing in the same area is elevated.

The high scorers on SOC and TSC/I are more than socially anxious; they tend also to be self-conscious, reserved, reticent, and show a tendency to withdraw under stress. At an intermediate elevated level they are introverted; at levels of T70 and above, schizoid.

Two other scales tap the opposite end of this dimension. One is Wiggins Hypomania Scale (HYP). Those scoring in the range T60–69 are outgoing individuals who usually appear cheerful and enthusiastic. Those with scores above T70 are likely to be easily excitable, impulsive, and emotionally labile, a condition that may reflect an immaturity that could interfere with the individual's productive existence.

One last scale that has some bearing on this dimension is the Harris and Lingoes Psychomotor Acceleration subscale (9PMA). 9PMA is a measure of the degree to which the individual requires sensation and excitement in his/her life; it is highly correlated with sensation-seeking. Normal adolescents and young adults, especially males, not infrequently score above T70 on this scale. Among adults in general, scores in the range T60–69 are associated with a tendency to extroversion, a lack of discomfort in social situations, and so on. Scores below T40 suggest discomfort and a tendency to withdraw.

SOME PERSONALITY PATTERNS REFLECTED
IN SPECIAL SCALE SCORES

Conforming and Moral

American moral standards are frequently violated by Americans. The statement is so manifestly true that it hardly seems cynical. There are also substantial numbers of people—primarily living in small towns and rural areas—who weigh moral values highly and who perceive themselves as moral, virtuous, and otherwise conforming to traditional cultural standards of personal behavior. They view the world unskeptically and believe that social malignancy and evil-doers are rare.

Such respondents elevate on 3NA and 6N primarily; sometimes on 5C, REL, and/or the Lie Scale. In fact, the conforming-moral pattern is the sole explanation of the high L Scale score in a person of normal intelligence. Negatively related scale scores are invariably low, especially 9AMO and including the alienation, hostility and suspicion scales especially E/Cy, Ho, and TSC/S.

This pattern is found mostly in adult women and need include only 3NA, 6N, and 9AMO. In such cases, the respondent is mainly claiming chastity for herself. When 5C and/or L are also elevated, the sexual morality is joined by affirmation of old-fashioned American virtues like honesty, trust, sportsmanship, and conservatism. When REL is also high, there is an evident spiritual basis for the respondent's pattern.

These respondents tend to deny anger and hostility and have low scores on HOS and TSC/R, occasionally an elevation on OH. The latter is one of the indicators of sincerity as opposed to denial in the conforming-moral person. T-scores above 70 on both 3NA and 6N and L scores over 10 suggest denial; the respondent needs to present him/herself as conforming and moral but does not demonstrate it behaviorally.

Authority Conflict

Rebelliousness is indicated by high scores on 4AC and AUT. Those scoring high on AUT appear to have some awareness of their difficulty in accepting the dictates of authority figures. High scorers on 4AC have a similar difficulty with restrictions and control but seem unaware of their rebellious findings.

The distinction in awareness of feelings between the two authority conflict scales is supported by the finding that it is not unusual for 4AC to elevate while AUT is within normal limits; the reverse is rare. The correlation between the two scales is only .30. Second, 4AC has substantial correlations with manifest hostility scales like HOS (.60), TSC/R (.49), and Ho (.76). AUT has minimal relationships with HOS (.28) and Ho (.17) and none with TSC/R.

Using adult norms, a number of normal adolescents, especially males, score in the range T65–70 on 4AC. TSC/R is sometimes also elevated. In delinquent adolescents, AUT, HOS, and Ho are also likely to be high.

Acting-Out

A high score on 9PMA ordinarily indicates a high optimum stimulation level. These individuals have a greater than normal need to have sensations, to experience excitement and will take risks to gain those experiences. They seek social, community, and sports activities and usually enjoy the company of others. The correlation of .79 with HYP is not unexpected (high 9PMA individuals low on HYP have a problem).

Scores of T60–70 are not uncommon among normal adolescents, especially males, and young adult males. Adolescents may even score above T70 without indicating serious psychopathology. However, when HOS or Ho are high, especially above T68, the prediction of hostile acting-out behavior is tenable. A potential for sexual acting-out may be inferred when Pe is above T65 in men or I-SP is elevated by either a male or female respondent.

Dependency–Dominance

Everyone has dependency and dominance needs. In most of us, the two are generally in balance and the net is unremarkable psychologically. Some individuals are overbalanced in one or the other need; such individuals are regarded as having a dependency or a dominance need that is psychologically notable. In the former instance, it is conventional to refer to a dependent personality. The consequence of a strong dominance need is not so clear since people who need to be dominant may or may not actualize that need successfully.

I-De and I-Do measure dependency need and dominance need, respectively. A respondent with I-De of T60 or above is usually classically dependent with self-esteem maintained largely extrinsically, lack of self-confidence, inability to make decisions, and a tendency to subordinate his/her needs and desires to the wishes of those on whom he/she depends. Such respondents rarely have scores on I-Do above T45 and never above T50.

Individuals with I-Do scores in the range T60–69 claim to be confident, self-assured, assertive, with strong opinions and a need to dominate relationships. Scores on I-De are seldom above T45 and are usually T40 and below.

Scores above T70 on I-Do suggest that the various claims of confidence, and the like, are probably not valid. This individual seeks urgently to be dominant in interpersonal spheres but lacks the necessary positive personality characteristics to succeed.

In the mid ranges of scores on I-De and I-Do, dependency and dominance needs are usually balanced and no diagnostic statement is required. Typically, the difference between the T-scores of the two scales will not exceed +10. In some cases, the interpretation of a scale depends on the level of the other. When either I-De is above T50 and I-Do is at least T15 less, a dependency need is manifested. Similarly, if I-Do is above T50 and I-De is at least T15 less, a statement concerning dominance is warranted. These are, of course, tendencies and are not stated as definitely as when scores reach T60.

Table 5.1 presents a young male exhibitionist who can best be described as passive–dependent, suggestible, and easily manipulated. He has serious problems relating to others, is shy, embarrasses easily in social situations, and has a marked tendency to withdraw into passivity in the face of stress. The elevations on Pe and I-SP are markers that indicate his sexual deviancy. Note that the hostility scales, HOS, Ho, and TSC/R, are all below normal and might have been expected to be even lower.

Passive–Aggressive

Dependent people need to think of themselves as agreeable and friendly; angry feelings are characteristically denied. One cannot afford hostility if one depends on others to assume one's responsibilities, make one's decisions and generally guide one's life. Thus, respondents who are judged to be dependent based on I-De and I-Do typically have low scores on hostility scales such as HOS, AUT, and Ho, like the case in Table 3.6.

We know that dependent people do harbor angry feelings and that some of them are characterized by a passive expression of that hostility in procrastination, forgetfulness, and sluggish behavior. Such individuals are often identified by scores of T60 or higher on some hostility scales, usually 4AC and/or TSC/R accompanying the I-De—I-Do imbalance that indicates the dependent person.

The Assertive Woman

The woman who scores T65 or above on Astvn is likely to be aware of her personal rights and to know something about the difference between assertiveness and aggression—but not invariably. Women with high scores on Astvn rarely have high scores on I-De—the correlation is −.51, an understandable finding. Neither do they tend to have scores above T60 on I-Do; the correlation is minimal .30. Rather, they fall into the group that ranges from T40 to T59 with I-Do higher than I-De.

A critical score is FEM which is unrelated to Astvn. Respondents with scores in the normal range of FEM are the appropriately assertive women. Those with low scores on FEM, especially lower than T40, are more likely to be aggressive rather than assertive and to give indications of rejecting a feminine gender identity. Not infrequently, I-SP will be elevated; examination of the items in this scale

TABLE 5.1
Young Adult Male Exhibitionist
Some Significant Scale Findings (T-Scores)

I-De	I-Do	TSC/I	SOC
60	15	69	72
HOS	TSC/R	Ho	TSC/S
42	45	45	39
	Pe	I-SP	
	64	75	

may reveal deviant responses to item 74 ("I have never been sorry that I am a girl"), and/or item 470 ("Sexual things disgust me").

The hostility scales are also relevant. TSC/R has a small, negative correlation (−.26) with Astvn. The other hostility scales are unrelated. The assertive woman who does not have a problem with gender identity will usually have hostility scales within the normal range. Elevations on the hostility scales are another indicator of the woman who is having a gender identity problem.

THE PERSONALITY DISORDERS[11]

Many of the diagnostic categories currently in use in the mental health field derive from florid symptoms such as anxiety, depression, guilt, and disorders of thought. Persons with neurotic or psychotic disorders hypothetically may, with appropriate treatment, become non-neurotic or nonpsychotic. In any event, some degree of restabilization or reduction of symptom severity can be accomplished in most cases. The obvious analogy being made is to physical diseases.

The entities that make up a major part of Axis II of the multiaxial DSM series (-III, -III-R, -IV) (American Psychiatric Association, 1980, 1987, 1994, respectively)—i.e., the personality disorders—are regarded differently. They are considered to be based on personality traits and behaviors that are more enduring than symptoms. Their roots can be traced to the developmental period, with the personality pattern emerging in adolescence or the early adult years. Thereafter, they are likely to be present all throughout the remainder of adult life. Personality

---

[11]Special thanks are due to Dr. James M. Schuerger for sharing with us unpublished correlational data between proposed MCMI and MMPI personality disorder scales (Millon, 1983; Morey, Blashfield, Webb, & Jewell, 1988) and an extensive array of MMPI special scales. These data helped to formulate some of the interpretive criteria in this section.

disorders are pervasive in scope, being interwoven with and affecting nearly all important aspects of the person's life. These special constellations of traits and behaviors result in either psychological distress or in impairment of functioning in social relations and occupational life.

A personality disorder may be conceptualized as a pattern of traits that have become intensified or exaggerated to the point of being dysfunctional. Traits themselves may be consequences of the specialized use of defense or coping strategies that develop relatively early in life for dealing with stress. Table 5.2 is a theoretical-logical illustration of relationships between defense mechanisms and personality characteristics and disorders, suggested by Levitt and Waddell (in press). Millon (1987) now links varying defense styles with each disorder as one of the eight criterial attributes used for classification.

The original MMPI clinical scales imply that the instrument was intended to measure clinical syndromes and not personality disorders. Subsequent research has, nevertheless, made it abundantly clear that the MMPI item pool is equal to measuring far more than was called for by the nosology of its time (Dahlstrom & Welsh, 1960; Dahlstrom et al., 1972, 1975). Yet attempts to bring MMPI items to bear on the specific DSM-based personality categories have been few (e.g., Morey, Waugh, & Blashfield, 1985; Zarrella, Schuerger, & Ritz, 1990). There seems in fact to be a studied avoidance of this issue in recent work of the team that undertook the development of MMPI-2 (Butcher, Dahlstrom, Graham, Tellegen, & Kaemmer, 1989; Graham, 1987, 1990). On a similar note, one of the central personality researchers who is very closely associated with Axis II personality disorder formulations from DSM-III through -IV (Millon, 1981) has bypassed this issue by developing instead his own inventory while dismissing the MMPI as a possible source of either items and special scales (Millon, 1983, 1987). The absence of borrowing or intellectual stimulation across the MMPI-2 and MCMI-II developer teams is too patently obvious to be attributed to inadvertent oversight. Unfortunately it has deprived the field of personality diagnosis of a potentially rich source of intellectual cross-fertilization.

The present effort is based on the considered belief that both MMPI items and special scales have relevance for measuring Axis II disorders within the

TABLE 5.2

Theoretical Relationships Between Defense Mechanisms,
Personality Traits and Personality Disorders

Defense Mechanism	Traits	Personality Disorder
Projection	Critical, intolerant, hostile	Paranoid
Regression	Dependent, demanding, irresponsible	Dependent
Repression	Inhibited, withdrawn, guarded	Schizoid
Compulsivity	Rigid, orderly, narrow, ruminative	Obsessive-Compulsive

DSM series. A number of special scales tap into personality characteristics rather than symptomology per se, as seen in Chapter 5, and are thus potentially useful for diagnosing personality disorders.

The personality disorders themselves are prototype entities rather than discrete categories. That is, they are more akin to oblique factors than to orthogonal solutions. This reality emerges because their developmental and life space experiential origins intermesh and are multifactorially determined. The result is a fair amount of overlap among the various personality disorders.

This overlap is acknowledged in DSM-III-R: ". . . to find a single, specific Personality Disorder that adequately describes the person's disturbed personality functioning. Frequently this can be done only with difficulty since many people exhibit traits that are not limited to a single Personality Disorder" (APA, 1987, p. 336). Additional acknowledgment is furnished by the cluster system of DSM-III-R in which disorders with similar traits are arranged in three groups.

Because of this overlap, MMPI special scales must be supplemented by use of specific MMPI item sets. Item sets can be selected in consideration of DSM criteria that are underrepresented by the special scales. This scales-plus-items approach to the diagnosis of personality disorders is followed in this volume. The next two sections of this chapter identify the special scales that are diagnostically applicable to each personality disorder and describe the methodology of selecting the individual items that supplement the scales. To avoid redundancy, the items themselves are presented only in Table 5.4.

Antisocial Personality Disorder. Several scales pertain to the sociopathic personality (Chapter 4). These individuals are irritable, angry, aggressive, and externalize their conflicts (high HOS and TSC/R). Their pervasive disregard for others' rights is based in an amoral outlook (high 9AMO; low 3NA and 6N) and, furthermore, in a correlated complex of mistrust, cynicism, and rationalization for misconduct (high Ho, E/Cy, TSC/S). They harbor a domineering attitude that makes it rare for them to tolerate well the normal frustrations of living (high I-Do and I-Do > I-De). The foregoing attitudes, coupled with low frustration tolerance, potentiate an inherent tendency toward impulsivity (high HYP and 9PMA). Their acting out potential is also increased by the disinhibiting effects of substance abuse (a higher tendency than other personality disorders to abuse street drugs, with this being superimposed on alcohol abuse). All of the foregoing results in authority conflict (high AUT and 4AC), social alienation (high 4SOA and 8SOA), and family difficulties (high FAM and 4FD).

The general pattern of antisocial special scales appears also in the paranoid personality disorder. What distinguishes antisocials are higher levels of: amorality, poor frustration tolerance, impulsivity and drug abuse seen among them. Moreover, conduct disordered action is another distinctive. Conduct disordered behavior is covered in the supplementary MMPI item set (Table 5.4), since the special scales do not include this aspect of their makeup and life history. Additional differences will be examined in the following section.

Paranoid Personality Disorder. These persons resemble antisocials in their pattern for: irritability, anger and externalization; mistrust, cynicism, and amorality (not quite so high 9AMO); domineering attitude; impulsive reactivity (somewhat less prominent); drug abuse (not quite as marked); authority conflict; social alienation; and family problems. Two additional features are more obviously distinguishing. They are exquisitely hypersensitive, feeling painfully exposed to emotional slight or injury (high 6P). Second, they go beyond mistrust into the zone of ominous suspiciousness of others (high S+). These latter two characteristics account for their behavior relative to a majority of the DSM criteria for this disorder (see Chapter 4 in this connection). The same traits may cause other psychotic indicators to elevate, but these are usually not nearly so high as those of psychotics—and they further are not accompanied in this disorder by psychotic signs of cognitive decompensation. Hence, this disorder is not easily confused with the psychoses. See also the related supplementary item set (Table 5.4).

Narcissistic Personality Disorder. The MMPI special scales profile for narcissists closely resembles that of histrionics. Their similarities will be reviewed first, since these set them apart from the other personality disorders. The need to be admired as well as profuse fantasies of impressing others appear on the special scales as claims of exceptional poise or social ease (very low SOC and TSC/I with very high 3DSA, 4SI, and 9IMP). No other disorders come close to narcissists and histrionics in this respect. Nevertheless, they do not claim to be particularly extroverted (average HYP). Not surprisingly, neither of these disorders is much interested in receiving intimate support from others (average 3NA) nor do they express a particularly trusting attitude (average 6N). For narcissists, the DSM criteria recognize the preceding in terms of their lacking empathy and viewing interpersonal contacts as sparking jealousy in one or both parties.

Narcissists and histrionics both express, further, a need to be in control of situations (I-Do > I-De). In connection with this, they see themselves as less emotionally vulnerable than most other personality disorders (slightly low 6P). For narcissists the foregoing are expressions of their exploitative style of relating. Finally, both disorders present themselves in hypernormal fashion, with consequent reduction of a broad range of symptomatic indicators (low ME). For narcissists, low ME also signals the underlying grandiose sense of self-importance and belief in their being "unique" and entitled to special treatment. Because of the substantial similarity of their profiles to those of histrionics, the supplementary item sets for these disorders (Table 5.4) often can play an essential role in telling them apart.

Histrionic Personality Disorder. Four fundamental special scale cluster markers of the histrionic's makeup are presented above relative to narcissists. The psychological implications of the clusters are, on the other hand, necessarily different. Histrionics' expressions of ease and poise in social situations correspond to their intense need to be the center of attention and lead also to their distorted perception that their relations with others are more intimate than they actually are. Relationships remain superficial, because attention rather than true intimacy is the goal and also because their feelings for others typically are shallow and shifting. Unlike narcissists, feelings of being in control do not so much indicate exploitative intent as they do histrionics' urgent desire to assure that they will remain at center stage. Hypernormal self perception ties in to the same need system, providing means of negating the symptomatic qualities that would be unattractive.

Because interactions with others are often inappropriately laden with erotic expression or provocative behavior, they experience difficulties in this area that distinguish them from narcissists: they are likely to have a sexual problem (elevated I-SP or, for males only, high Pe). Their excessively impressionistic manner of speech indicates an underlying cognitive style that may be reflected on special scales as unsystematic, fragmented thinking (high TR + CLS) that cannot be explained by either limited intellect or poor reading comprehension. The supplementary item set (Table 5.4) should also be considered in establishing this diagnosis.

Borderline Personality Disorder.   Borderlines present with overall elevated MMPI special scale patterns, as do also passive aggressives, avoidants, and schizotypals (i.e., all having increased ME to varying extents, with multiple content scales elevated). Borderlines, however, present a special scale profile that shares many similarities with that of passive aggressives, while distinguishing them both from avoidants and schizotypals. These profile distinctives include the presence of at least mild extroversion (elevated HYP) in borderlines coupled with unusually mixed indicators of social maladjustment (average scores on SOC and TSC/I, lowered 3DSA, 4SI and 9IMP, elevated 6P). They have mild authority conflict (mildly elevated AUT), family difficulty (high FAM and 4FD), and marked anxiety (high TSC/T). Finally, they seek excitement (elevated 9PMA) and appear to have adequate energy (average 2PR). Borderlines share the foregoing distinctives with passive aggressives, although their levels differ on particular scale clusters. Avoidants and schizotypals do not have this pattern of characteristics, as will be further emphasized in their respective sections.

Borderlines differ from passive aggressives by having notably higher mean elevation (ME) and elevations on as many as 20 special scales, reflecting the wide variety of symptoms that they experience (see Chapter 2). Affective symptoms of all types (e.g., HOS, DEP, TSC/T) and poor self image (high MOR, I-SC, and 2MD) account for the most prominent of these content scale elevations in borderlines. Their affective symptoms in particular elevate greatly during crisis periods, at which times they may also exhibit paranoid (high S+) or dissociative (I-DS) signs. As an example of their affective profile, borderlines are set apart from passive aggressives by having more marked social anxiety (lower 3DSA, etc., as noted above) and greater sensitivity (higher 6P), while borderlines' SOC and TSC/I are average—somewhat higher for passive aggressives.

Regarding the last cluster noted above, borderlines are especially distinctive in the extent to which the usual negative relationship disappears between SOC and the triad of social anxiety scales (e.g., 3DSA, etc.). Thus, they do not retreat from the considerable interpersonal turmoil that they experience—an indication of their extreme need to pursue idealized relationships or avoid abandonment. Borderlines display another special scale pattern that departs from what is typically seen: they combine elevated HYP and DEP which are usually negatively related. Their unusual mixture of HYP and DEP, coupled with 9PMA and 2PR, relate to the DSM criteria of affective instability and to impulsive actions that proceed from this. Borderlines, further, are notably prone to abuse both drugs and alcohol (high AMac)—tendencies that are not remarkable among passive aggressives. They are of course known for their prominent suicidal and self-injurious behaviors which also distinguish them from passive aggressives. Additional differences from passive aggressives are considered in the following section. The supplementary MMPI personality disorder item set (Table 5.4) may also be useful for differentiating these two groups.

Passive Aggressive Personality Disorder.   Several similarities and differences between passive aggressives and borderlines can be found in the preceding section, where selected guidelines are presented for differentiating between them. See also the earlier discussion of some marker traits and special scales for the measurement of passive aggressiveness.

Passive aggressives feel externally controlled (high E/Cy) and powerless (I-De > I-Do). Consequently they feel unable to exercise the initiative needed to help themselves (high 8CON). This is accompanied by markedly poor self image (high MOR, I-SC and 2MD), as is true of borderlines, but without the signs of depression that usually accompany this (i.e., average DEP, TSC/D, etc.). Because of their social contrariness they feel socially anxious and awkward (same pattern of 3DSA, 4SI, 9IMP, and 6P as borderlines but with elevations also of SOC and TSC/I). Contrary aspects of the passive aggressive condition are also displayed by resentment that exceeds hostility (TSC/R > HOS, both scales elevated) and rebelliousness of which they have only very limited awareness (AUT > 4AC, with 4AC being only average). With this comes anxiety about retaliation from others (high TSC/T) for their contrariness. All of this leaves them feeling socially alienated (elevated 4SOA and 8SOA). They tend to blame family members for failing to satisfy their dependency needs (high FAM and 4FD). See also Table 5.4 for the supplementary item set that touches on aspects of this disorder.

Dependent Personality Disorder.   This disorder little resembles others, except for some similarity to compulsives and passive aggressives. Its first distinctive is very marked dependency (I-De > I-Do). In females this will also appear as low assertiveness (Astvn). At all costs dependents avoid challenging authority (low AUT and 4AC). In fact, they are so needy that they cannot express hostility openly (low HOS), although they may express adolescent type resentment (elevated

TSC/R). Expressions of mistrust and cynicism are accordingly low (low Ho, E/Cy and TSC/S). Dependents also display low self confidence (high MOR and I-SC) and strong feelings of personal inadequacy (high 2MD and 8COG). Negative self feelings contribute to low energy and attainment, helping maintain their defect of initiative (high 2PR and 8CON with low HYP and 9PMA). Their avoidance of challenging authority or of expressing hostility correlates with their feelings of safety in conventionality (high 5C). Their attempts to submit, avoid offending others, and otherwise to be deferential, nevertheless, fail to ward off concerns that their dependency needs will not be met. Thus, they experience either anxiety (high TSC/T) or depression (high DEP, 2SD, TSC/D) fairly constantly in response to real or imagined threats to their dependency. Due to poor self image and their nagging concerns over loss of support, dependents are hypersensitive and vulnerable in interpersonal relationships (high 6P). The supplementary item set (Table 5.4) and the earlier discussion of the dependent personality in this chapter can aid in identifying this disorder.

Obsessive Compulsive Personality Disorder. As the DSM criteria make clear, the principal traits of this disorder relate more to compulsivity than to being obsessional. For this reason, elevations on the I-OC scale are not expected; I-OC instead is expected with the neurosis, that is now designated obsessive compulsive disorder, or other serious disturbances (see Chapter 3). Only occasionally does the neurosis appear as a co-morbid condition with this personality disorder. Chapter 5 covers the conformity-morality cluster that is most central to the compulsive's makeup.

Among their distinctives, compulsives elevate on 3NA and 6N and receive very low scores on 9AMO, E/Cy, Ho, and TSC/S. Along with these they manifest high conventionality (high 5C). Their need to feel tightly in control of themselves is expressed by the following: a dominant attitude (I-Do > I-De); the belief that they can behave constructively (8CON) and with emotions closely controlled (low HYP); the illusion of fitting in socially (low SOC and TSC/I along with elevated 3DSA, 4SI, and 9IMP) but with surprisingly low vulnerability to what others think of them (low 6P); and a determined stance not to become venturesome or overstimulated (low 9PMA). Their low HYP and 9PMA are not associated with a deficit of energy (average 2PR).

They deny symptomatic and socially conflictual or negative traits with greater consistency than is true for any other personality disorder. An exception to this is that somatic complaints often are not viewed as forbidden (potential for elevated HEA and TSC/B). Extensive denial results in very low mean elevation (ME) of basic clinical scales and correspondingly low scores on pertinent special scales. Not uncommonly they register raw scores of zero on multiple special scales. This self-enhancing perspective results from a reigning perfectionism. Notable examples of hypernormal scores are those for social alienation (low 4SOA and 8SOA) and social hypersensitivity (low 6P), for both of which they receive on average the lowest scores of any personality disorder. Hostile feelings are also among the most strongly denied or repressed (very low HOS and TSC/R). Nevertheless, in especially conflictual situations, the rigor of their defensiveness leads to overcontrolled hostility (OH > HOS and TSC/R). At such times their coping style assumes the obsessional quality of a reaction formation, including determined externalization of responsibility (e.g., AUT elevates—normally being low), and feelings of tension rise precipitously (high TSC/T—normally low). Thus obsessive compulsives seek by externalization to preserve intact a hypernormal self image. The supplementary item set (Table 5.4) can be helpful in initial identification of this disorder.

Avoidant Personality Disorder.   Avoidant, schizotypal, and schizoid personality disorders share a common core that differentiates them from the other eight disorders. This core is comprised of extreme social discomfort or anxiety (very low 3DSA, 4SI, and 9IMP) together with the correlated tendency to withdraw into isolation or avoid social contact under stress (very high SOC and TSC/I). The Avoidant-Schizotypal-Schizoid Core supplementary item set (Table 5.4) captures the essentials of the foregoing special scale cluster, including also relevant items that appear in none of the foregoing special scales. Schizoids can next be distinguished from the other two disorders by use of the Avoidant-Schizotypal Core supplementary set. Schizoids score low on this scale due to their flat affectivity. Both avoidants and schizotypals score high because they experience a chronic dysphoric, mixed type of emotional reactivity that also elevates special scales (high DEP, 2SD, TSC/D, TSC/T and mildly elevated HOS), all of which set these two types apart from schizoids. Congruently, they suffer from poor morale and self-esteem (high MOR and I-SC) which are decidedly less marked in schizoids. These are among the many scale elevations that result in high mean elevation (high ME) for avoidants and schizotypals but not for schizoids.

Markers that differentiate between avoidants and schizotypals appear within the mix of multiple elevations that raise ME. Specifically, avoidants have even more extreme scores on the social discomfort/anxiety and withdrawal scales than do schizotypals (see preceding paragraph). These scale elevations relate to avoidants' pervasive social inhibition and hypersensitivity to the potential for others to criticize or reject them. Avoidants further express stronger doubts about the reliability of their mental processes and their ability to function (very high 2MD, 8COG, and 8CON). This cluster meshes with the DSM criteria which recognize that they feel inept, unappealing, inadequate, inferior, and at constant risk of embarrassing themselves with resultant humiliation and rejection. The supplementary Avoidant item set (Table 5.4) samples additional perspectives on this disorder.

Schizotypal Personality Disorder.   Many of the distinctive signs of the presence of this disorder have already been discussed in the context of the avoidant disorder, which it resembles in several respects. Thus, the section on avoidant personality should be closely consulted for both similarities and differences. The most distinctive marker of schizotypal personality is the prominence of psychotic indicators within the overall elevated profile. Rather than the avoidant's fear of rejection and embarrassment, the social anxiety of schizotypals tends to relate to paranoid suspicions and fears along with ideas of reference (high 6PI, PSY, and S+). Their proneness to unusual percepts, including somatic illusions, may also be reflected in special scales (high ORG, I-DS, 8BSE, I-RD). Under stress, more frankly psychotic experiences may occur with this disorder. Additional perspectives on this disorder are captured by the supplementary item set for Schizotypal (Table 5.4).

Schizoid Personality Disorder. The detection of schizoids by a systematic process of eliminating alternatives is presented in the Avoidant section, which should be consulted in this regard. Although they share social discomfort and withdrawal with the two preceding disorders, their social sensitivity is not remarkable (average 6P). They show little of the emotional distress or hostility seen in their counterparts—an indication of their detachment and flattened affectivity. Along with this, they have low energy (high 2PR) and do not desire to raise their level of arousal (average 9PMA). They seem unconcerned about their lack of connectedness (fairly average 4SOA and 8SOA). Unlike their counterparts, ME is fairly average as well. They are notable for their use of drugs in particular and also alcohol (elevated AMac), which sets them apart from avoidants and schizotypals. No supplementary item set could be constructed from MMPI items beyond the index of withdrawal and social discomfort that they share with avoidants and schizotypals. Nevertheless, the constellation of special scales noted above plus schizoids' similarity on the Avoidant-Schizotypal-Schizoid Core and dissimilarity on the Avoidant-Schizotypal Core (Table 5.4) make it possible to differentiate them from avoidants and schizotypals.

Table 5.3 summarizes salient special scale levels for each of the personality disorders by presenting all the essential relationships in schematic coded form. Minimal relationships are indicated by + or −. Strong relationships are assigned multiple pluses and minuses. Scales that are uncorrelated with disorders are identified by a zero but only if the absence of relationship is diagnostically significant. Disorders appear in the table as columns in the order of their treatment in the preceding text. The special scales are in rows in the order of their employment in Appendix V. Usually, the scales are entered as clusters unless the scales within a cluster relate to the disorder with varying degrees of strength in which case they will be found in separate rows within the table.

Personality Disorder Items: Selection Procedure

All 550 items were studied individually in relation to the listed DSM-III-R criteria plus Millon's criteria (Millon, 1987) for each of the 11 personality disorders.[12]

---

[12]DSM-III-R (APA, 1987) was our reference document for the selection of items because DSM-IV (APA, 1994) was not yet available. DSM-IV determined the choice of scales, following the preliminary publication of this document (APA, 1993).

TABLE 5.3
Profile Characteristics Differentiating Among Personality Disorders

Special Scales	Personality Disorders										
	ANTI	PRND	NARC	HIST	BORD	P-AG	DPND	OB-C	AVDT	SZTY	SCZD
TR, CI				++							
ME			−	−		+		− −	+++	+++	0
DEP, etc.				+1	++	0	+2		++	++	
MOR, I-SC					++	++	++		+++	+++	
Suicidal					++1						
TSC/T					++	+	+2	++1	++	++	
I-DS, etc.				+1	+1					++	
PSY, etc.		+								++	
S+		+			+1					++	
8COG, 2MD	+++	+++			+	0, +	++	− −	+++	++	
8CON	++	++				++	++	− − −	+++	++	++
HOS	+++				++	+	− −	− −	+	+	
TSC/R	++				+	+++	+2	− −	+	+	
OH > HOS, etc.								++1			
HEA, TSC/B								+2			
3DSA, etc.			++	++	− −	−		++	− − −	− −	− −
SOC, TSC/I			− −	− −	0	+	−	−	+++	++	+++
HYP	++	+	0	0	++	+	−	−		++	−
9PMA	+++	+			++	+		− −			−

(Continued)

85

TABLE 5.3
(Continued)

Personality Disorders

Special Scales	ANTI	PRND	NARC	HIST	BORD	P-AG	DPND	OB-C	AVDT	SZTY	SCZD
2PR			−	−	0		+	0	++		++
6P	++	+++	−	−	++	+	+	−−	++	++	0
4SOA, 8SOA		+++						−−	+	+	0
AUT	+++	+++			+	++	−	−, +1			
4AC	++	++			+	0	−	−, +1			
Ho, etc.	+++	+++				E/Cy+	−−	−−			
I-De	−−	−−	−			+	++	−			
I-Do, Astvn	+++	++	+			−−	−−, −3	+			
FAM, 4FD	++	++			++	++			+		0
AMac					++	0					
Drugs	+++	++			++2	0					++
I-SP, Pe				++, +4							
3NA, 6N	−−	−−	0	0				++			
9AMO	+++	++					++	−−			
5C	−−	−−						+++			

Key: (+) = above average; (0) = average; (−) = below average. Note that zeroes (0) are entered only when referenced in text as contrasts or unusual.
1 Crisis indicator
2 Possible sign; not inconsistent if present but need not be
3 Females only
4 Males only

TABLE 5.4

Items for the Diagnosis of Personality Disorders

Disorder	True	False
Antisocial	49/66, 56/84, 93/81, 118/105, 124/110, 135/123, 145/134, 146/156, 205/240, 218/270, 250/227, 269/324, 271/248, 298/269, 313/283, 381/389, 419/412, 437/418, 471/431, 472/432, 475/433	37/34, 113/126, 294/266
Paranoid	16/17, 28/27, 35/42, 110/99, 136/124, 157/145, 162/151, 200/228, 247/300, 265/241, 278/251, 284/259, 303/274, 348/315, 364/333, 448/424, 507/445	79/63, 347/314
Narcissistic	19/19, 24/22, 35/42, 73/61, 122/109, 165/153, 247/300, 257/318, 264/239, 271/248, 280/254, 282/256, 299/271, 317/285, 336/302, 353/321, 400/345, 411/347, 415/350, 417/410, 469/358, 511/448, 521/262	86/73, 198/184
Histrionic	22/23, 25/25, 126/112, 158/146, 181/169, 248/226, 266/242, 336/302, 353/321, 381/389, 386/393, 482/342, 506/444, 521/262, 555/469	171/158, 180/167, 240/220, 262/237, 304/275, 306/278, 312/281, 407/405
Borderline	22/23, 39/37, 61/52, 67/56, 74/62 (male), 75/102, 94/82, 104/92, 129/116, 139/150, 145/134, 158/146, 208/189, 234/213, 236/215, 299/271, 301/273, 305/277, 381/389, 383/338, 418/411, 468/430, 506/444, 555/469	8/9, 37/34, 74/62 (female), 379/388, 399/472, 407/405
Passive-Aggressive	13/15, 41/38, 109/98, 157/145, 212/190, 233/212, 244/225, 245/288, 259/233, 342/308, 487/364, 536/461	83/108, 96/83
Dependent	82/70, 86/73, 141/129, 259/233, 357/326, 394/398, 398/348, 443/421, 531/457, 549/368, 564/369	46/43, 73/61, 112/120, 122/109, 170/157, 228/206, 235/214, 257/318, 371/335, 501/440, 520/452
Obsessive-Compulsive	64/55, 112/120, 148/136, 213/193, 232/211, 233/212, 343/309, 346/313, 359/328, 390/396, 404/403, 427/351, 431/415, 461/356, 499/442, 558/470	None
Avoidant	86/73, 138/127, 191/178, 267/243, 301/273, 304/275, 305/277, 321/289, 344/310, 368/386, 382/390, 509/446	79/63, 187/177, 371/335, 521/262
Schizotypal	27/24, 33/32, 50/72, 110/99, 121/138, 136/124, 265/241, 284/259, 293/361, 345/311, 348/315, 349/316, 364/333, 551/466	450/359, 464/427, 482/392
Schizoid[a] Avoidant-Schizotypal Core	180/167, 278/251, 317/285	170/157, 230/208, 353/321, 407/405
Avoidant-Schizotypal-Schizoid Core	52/46, 292/265, 312/281, 377/337, 384/391, 473/367	54/78, 57/49, 309/280, 440/354, 449/353, 451/363, 479/360, 547/370

Note. Original MMPI item number listed first followed by MMPI-2 number.

[a]Schizoid Personality Disorder is diagnosed indirectly from a comparison of the Avoidant-Schizotypal core and the Avoidant-Schizotypal-Schizoid core. Schizoids will respond in the pathological direction to more items on the latter core than the former, possibly Level III or IV compared to Level I or II (see Table 5.5).

Thus, in each complete pass through the MMPI, items were selected to comprise a list for only one disorder. Each selected item was further coded to identify the criterion or criteria of DSM-III-R with which it was associated from a content validity perspective. A preference was given to items appearing also in MMPI-2. The 11 newly formed lists were then compared to the 11 lists of Morey et al. (1985) which had been assembled earlier to represent the criteria of DSM-III. Their items were all drawn from the original MMPI, since MMPI-2 had not yet been published. Matches were noted between the two sets of lists. There were also numbers of items appearing in only one or the other set of lists, creating a potential to increase the number of items in each of the 11 item pools while enhancing criterial match.

Following the preliminary inspection mentioned above, the two sets of lists were randomly merged to mask their respective origins, with one merged list per personality disorder. Each merged list appeared on a single two-column page. A cover page was placed on each list containing uniform instructions for evaluating items for goodness of match to DSM criteria. Pertinent sets of DSM-III-R criteria for the 11 disorders were then listed below the instructions for each personality group, yielding one cover sheet per disorder. The instructions called for marking the numbers of the items in a particular manner to indicate whether each item matched any of the listed criteria, a combination of them or the disorder's general description—or whether it matched none of these. Instructions stated that unmarked items should be understood as keyed true; all items keyed false were marked "F."

Eight judges independently reviewed each of the 11 merged item lists, marking items per the instructions. All were clinically experienced in use of the MMPI and DSM-III-R. Five were Ph.D. level psychologists, two were predoctoral interns, and one was a master's level clinician with extensive experience.

All sets of judgments were reviewed for completeness. If any items appeared to be overlooked, the judge was contacted and asked to make a definitive choice. Items agreed upon by at least seven judges were automatically retained in their respective item pools, except that if they were unavailable in MMPI-2 they were usually deleted. If only six of eight judges agreed, other factors were considered in deciding whether to retain the item—e.g., judged need for items to represent undersampled DSM criteria, probability that the item would discriminate between normals and relevant clinic cases based on contemporary item endorsement norms when available. If five or fewer judges agreed, the item was dropped.

The product of this effort was an update and content analysis cross-validation of the Morey et al. (1985) item lists, on which considerable research has been conducted since 1985, for example, Dubro, Wetzler, and Kahn (1988), Morey, Blashfield, Webb, and Jewell (1988), Morey and Smith (1988), Zarella et al. (1990).

As we noted in the discussion of scales in this section (pp. 83–84), the symptom overlap between Schizoid Personality Disorder and Avoidant and Schizotypal Personality Disorders makes it unfeasible to diagnose Schizoid Personality Dis-

TABLE 5.5

Frequencies of Endorsed Personality Disorder Items Corresponding to Levels of Disorder

	Level									
	I		II		III		IV		V	
Disorder	Male	Female	Male	Female	Male	Female	Male	Female	Male	Female
Antisocial	10	8	11	10	12	11	13	12	15	14
Paranoid	9	9	10	11	11	12	12	14	14	17
Narcissistic	13	12	14	14	15	15	16	16	18	19
Histrionic	11	12	12	13	13	14	14	15	15	17
Borderline	14	16	16	18	17	20	19	23	22	27
Passive-Aggressive	7	7	8	9	8–9	10	9	11	11	14
Dependent	10	11	11	13	12	14	13	16	15	19
Obsessive-Compulsive	8	9	9	10	10	11	11	13	13	15
Avoidant	7	8	8	10	9	11	11	13	13	16
Schizotypal	7	7	8	9	9	10	10	11	12	14
Avoidant-Schizotypal	4	4	5	5	5–6	6	6	7	7	–[a]
Avoidant-Schizotypal-Schizoid	6	6	8	7	9	8	10	10	13	12

Note: Level I = disorder is not present but a personality type is indicated.
　　　Level II = disorder is possibly present.
　　　Level III = disorder is probably present.
　　　Level IV = disorder is definitely present.
　　　Level V = disorder is very marked.
[a]The maximum score for Avoidant-Schizotypal is 7.

order directly. It is identified by a comparison of the Avoidant-Schizotypal-Schizoid core which it resembles closely and the Avoidant-Schizotypal core with which it has less in common. Thus, Table 5.4 which contains an update and expansion of the Morey et al. (1985) cross-validated item lists consists of 12 MMPI-2 compatible lists. This table and its collateral Table 5.5 are intended solely for the diagnosis of personality disorder and are not appropriate for the general assessment of personality.

Percentages of endorsements for each item in Table 5.4 are available for hospitalized psychiatric patient samples of 232 males and 191 females (Butcher et al., 1989). These percentages are easily converted into raw scores that permit the computation of mean scores for each personality disorder in Table 5.4. Unfortunately, Appendix I in Butcher et al. (1989) does not include variance data. We estimated standard deviations for the Butcher et al. distributions using a demographically similar local inpatient psychiatric sample. This sample consisted of 50 males and 50 females to whom the original MMPI had been administered and whose records met the validity standards in Section I of Appendix V. The standard deviations for the distributions of item sets for each personality disorder were then computed and converted into standard scores. Normal deviates could then be applied to create the levels of personality disorder in Table 5.5.

The norms in Table 5.5 are arranged in five columns headed by Roman numerals. Each numeral represents a percentile in the distribution of scores for our patient sample. Level I represents the 50 percentile. At this level, the respondent acknowledges a constellation of traits that is within normal limits. Level II scores (the 65th percentile) can be interpreted to mean that the disorder is *possibly* present. At Level III (the 75th percentile), the disorder is *probably* present. The interpretations of Levels IV and V, the 85th and 95th percentile respectively, leave little room for doubt that the disorder is *clearly* or *markedly* present. Thus, Levels II–V signify a personality or mixed personality disorder while Level I suggests a type of personality structure that is not psychopathological. Scores above Level V are usually secondary to Axis I disorders or may be a consequence of an elevated ME.

The data in Table 5.5 are suggestive but seldom conclusive. Diagnosis of personality disorder must be based not only on items but on the scale data summarized in Table 5.3 and the interpretive rules in Appendix V.

CHAPTER 6
MMPI SPECIAL SCALES
AND THE RORSCHACH[13]

Surveys over the years have shown that the MMPI and the Rorschach are two of the most frequently used diagnostic instruments in mental health facilities (Sundberg, 1961; Lubin, Larsen, & Matarazzo, 1983; Wade & Baker, 1977). The common assumption is that each measures psychopathology and taps personality trends but from a different direction, as might be expected of an objective and a projective test. A further assumption is that the MMPI draws on the respondent's conscious view of himself/herself while the Rorschach taps tendencies that exist below the level of the subject's conscious awareness. Thus, the common joint usage of these two instruments is understandable.

OVERVIEW OF THE EARLY
CORRELATIONAL STUDIES

In view of their popularity, one might expect that there would be considerable interest in the formal relationship between the MMPI and the Rorschach. Certainly appropriate correlational studies have the potential for many interesting findings that might have broad bearing on personality theory and psychopathology.

---

[13]The content of this chapter assumes a familiarity with the basics of Rorschach scoring and interpretation. The reader who is unfamiliar with the Rorschach might consult Exner (1993) or Levitt (1980a).

It is disappointing to discover that there have been only a handful of investigations into the relationship between the Rorschach and the MMPI over the past
decade, actually an average of about one a year. Eliminating the overlap from three
reviews of such studies (Levitt, 1989; Archer & Krishnamurthy, 1993a, 1993b),
the total is exactly 50. Thirty involved only the standard clinical and validity scales
and only a few special scales were included in the remaining reports, primarily
Barron's Ego-Strength scale, Taylor's Manifest Anxiety scale and Welsh's Anxiety
and Repression scales. Several reports (e.g., Smith & Coyle, 1969; Brems &
Johnson, 1990) indicate that a substantial number of special scales were included
in the analysis but they are not named.

Overall, the investigations of the relationship between the Rorschach and the
MMPI have been methodologically poor. Among the criticisms mentioned by
reviewers (Levitt, 1989; Archer & Krishnamurthy, 1993b) are small sample sizes,
variability or unclarity in administration and scoring of the Rorschach, no demonstration of scorer reliability, no statement of whether the Rorschach records
were obtained by a single examiner or by multiple examiners, and the source of
the records is unspecified.

No study of the relationship between Rorschach factors and the special scales
discussed in this book has yet been published. There are, however, two unpublished works which report intercorrelations between a large number of objective
Rorschach factors and many special scales.

The Reading and Haymond Theses

Correlational analyses not found in the published reports of relationships among
Rorschach data and MMPI special scales are available in two unpublished theses
(Haymond, 1981; Reading, 1978). These studies employed a standard Rorschach
administration procedure (Levitt, 1980a); all of the records were obtained and
scored by the same examiner and the MMPIs were scored for a large number of
special scales. The administrative standardization attempted to eliminate the examiner factor from the Rorschach data while the special scales made possible a
relatively wide variety of hypotheses.

Each study suffered from some unfortunate weaknesses, nevertheless. The
Reading study used only 25 subjects after discarding an unknown number because
the Rorschach inquiries were inadequate for scoring. In some cases, the MMPI
was given first, in others, the Rorschach.

The Haymond study had an N of 100 and none were discarded for any reason.
In every case, the MMPI was administered approximately 10 days prior to the
Rorschach. Haymond's sample, while respectable in size, is narrow in scope
since it was composed entirely of females between the ages of 12 and 18 who
had been referred to a juvenile diagnostic center. The sample had a mean IQ of
92 and the reading comprehension in the group required that the MMPI be
administered to some subjects by means of a cassette tape.

Despite the defects of these investigations they are worth examining.

Es did poorly in both investigations. Haymond found no relationship between Es and Rorschach measures of adjustment like F+%, XF+%, M, or FC. Reading reported a *positive correlation* between F– and Es and a *negative relationship* between F+ and Es.

Earlier investigations had hinted at the possibility that Rorschach content rather than formally scored factors might be more related to MMPI scales. This turned out to be the case to some extent in the Reading thesis. Two such Rorschach factors had understandable correlations with a large number of MMPI special scales. They were *perseveration* and *sex content*. Perseveration is the senseless repetition of a response through the Rorschach card deck; in Exner terms, content perseveration (Exner, 1993).

> The match between the shape of the object and the shape of the blot is fairly accurate when the response is first given; when the response is repeated in subsequent cards, however, the form of the blot is forced into the form of the object, in almost complete disregard of the actual form properties of the blots, the object, or both. (Klopfer & Spiegelman, 1956, p. 285)

While perseveration is regarded as a sign of serious psychopathology—schizophrenia or organic brain damage—sex content is usually thought of as a reflection of anxiety and a neurotic adjustment (Goldfried, Stricker, & Weiner, 1971). Beck, for example, considered Sx (the number of responses with sex as content) as an indicator of free-floating anxiety although he also suggested that it might reflect a serious regression (Beck, 1952).

In the Reading study, Sx had significant positive correlations ranging from .41 to .65 with 10 indices of psychopathology including I-RD, I-DS, PSY, and PHO; positive correlations ranging from .46 to .58 with seven measures of sociopathy such as Ho, HOS, and 4SOA. In addition, the obvious hypothesis of a relationship between Sx and I-SP was validated by a coefficient of .56.

The occurrence of perseveration had positive correlations ranging from .40 to .78 with six measures of psychopathology including I-RD and PSY and positive coefficients ranging from .43 to .57 with seven measures of sociopathy including Ho, 9AMO, and AMac. The obvious hypothesis of a relationship with I-OC was supported by a correlation coefficient of .55. It should be noted that the anatomy response, generally considered to be an indicator of psychopathology on the Rorschach, was unrelated to MMPI indices of psychopathology including most of the health concerns scales.

In the Haymond study, most of the significant correlation coefficients were between .20 and .30, fairly small compared to those in the Reading thesis. However, they are not unexpected in view of the homogeneity of Haymond's population. Among Haymond's data, Sx and perseveration do not stand out. They were totally unrelated to MMPI indices of psychopathology, mostly due to the fact that their means were very close to zero. Another Rorschach index of psychopathology—*contaminatory tendency*—was significantly positively related to seven MMPI psychopathology scales including I-RD and PSY. A contamination is the fusion of two incompatible objects into a single, peculiar, or bizarre percept. By unanimous clinical consensus, it is a hallmark of the schizophrenic respondent. A contaminatory tendency—what Exner (1993) calls an Inappropriate Combination—is a sort of minor contamination in that the alien objects are in different parts of the blot, such as "a person with the head of a chicken." Contaminatory tendency occurs in the Rorschach records of normal respondents but it occurs almost twice as often in the records of psychiatric outpatients and nearly four times as frequently in the records of psychiatric inpatients (Exner, 1991).

Haymond had some other interesting findings. For example, figure-ground reversal, usually considered to be a Rorschach indicator of negativism and hostility, was significantly related to HOS, AUT, and 9AMO. XF+%, generally considered to be the best indicator of adjustment on the Rorschach, had expected negative correlations with I-RD, I-DS, and 8BSE. The alienation scales 4SOA and 8SOA had significant negative relationships with H%, the percent of human responses in the Rorschach record, again not unexpectedly. Cn had a significant positive relationship with M, the number of movement responses, as might be expected from the clinical interpretation of Cn. Similarly, 5C has a significant relationship with P, the number of popular responses on the Rorschach, usually considered to be a mark of attunement to the demands of conventionality. As in the Reading thesis, the anatomy response was unrelated to MMPI measures of psychopathology including health concern scales.

Many of the hypotheses that were tested in the Reading and Haymond works were not supported by their data. However, there is enough in the way of positive findings, despite the methodological shortcomings of these studies, to suggest strongly that the Rorschach is supporting the validity of its old team mate—to use the metaphor employed in the title of Haymond's dissertation—at least insofar as special scales are concerned.

CONJOINT USE OF THE RORSCHACH AND THE MMPI

The MMPI and the Rorschach are commonly employed together in various clinical settings. The two instruments frequently complement each other to improve effectiveness and accuracy of assessment. The MMPI furnishes a greater variety of data on symptoms and personality traits. The Rorschach has the advantage of unfakability and thus has the capacity to distinguish between MMPI records that are the result of response sets and other misleading circumstances.

There is no shortage of cases, especially in forensic psychology, of faking bad MMPI records with an ME of T75 and greater that have companion Rorschach profiles that are clearly within normal limits. XF+% is between 75 and 90, *P* is at least 5 and pathological content and other qualitative indicators of a thought disorder are absent. Or, DEP and/or TSC/D are substantially elevated but the respondent pays no attention to the dark coloration in the blots. This anomaly is not unusual in a patient who is loudly proclaiming unhappiness and dissatisfaction with the current life space and is demanding help but is not clinically depressed.

On the other side of the coin, there are some seriously disturbed individuals who are able to exercise sufficient control when presented with a structured stimulus so that they produce minimally abnormal, or even normal, MMPI records. The amorphous ink blots, however, are likely to evoke unmistakable psychopathology. For example, $XF+\%$ and P may be low while the percentage of anatomy and sex responses may be high and qualitative indicators of thought disorder such as contamination, confabulation, loose associations, and bizarre content, may be present. Table 6.1 presents some contrasting MMPI and Rorschach data from the records of a 37-year-old white male inpatient whose only complaints were physical as evidenced by substantial elevations on TSC/B, ORG, and 8BSE. The patient was something of a medical mystery; his physical complaints had persisted over a number of years and were complicated by side effects of prescribed drugs.

Table 6.1 illustrates the absence of psychopathology in the MMPI record and the testimony to an underlying psychotic process by Rorschach data.

While the Rorschach is used not infrequently to correct a specious impression created by the MMPI, the two are also often used conjointly, either providing support for each other or complementary information. Three relevant case presentations follow.

The Case of DM

DM was a 27-year-old, white, married female with a high school education who had recently assumed a managerial position with a supermarket chain. She was referred to a Chronic Pelvic Pain Clinic operated by the Department of Obstetrics & Gynecology of a large metropolitan hospital. Typically, referrals were from physicians in the community in cases where multiple diagnostic procedures did not uncover an appropriate etiology for the patient's clinical symptoms.

TABLE 6.1
Conjoint Use of the MMPI and Rorschach

MMPI Data					Rorschach Data			
ME	PSY	I-RD	TSC/T	DEP	$XF+\%$	P	An%	Qualitative Signs
59	52	46	51	48	50	2	36	present

From records of a 37-year-old, white, male, inpatient, obtained 4 days apart. The qualitative signs of thought disorder on the Rorschach included vagueness, loose associations and confabulation.

Examination at the CPP Clinic disclosed a previously undiscovered organic basis for the presenting complaint in an occasional patient. The vast majority of the CPP clinic patients, however, turned out to have a psychogenic basis for their symptoms as evidenced by multiple minor physical complaints and emotional symptoms, especially problems of sexual identity or sexual function. Case DM was one of the few who did not fit the psychogenic pattern and medical staff were advised to look further for organic causes. Eventually, a previously unde-tected tumor was found and removed.

Three years later, the lady was referred to the Psychiatry Department at another metropolitan hospital by the Rheumatology Department, needing to find some reason for persistent and progressive pains described as polyarthralgias and chronic right-sided weakness. On the occasion of this admission, a Rorschach was added to the MMPI.

What follows is a point-by-point description of the conjoint interpretation of the Rorschach and the MMPI. Note especially that both instruments are required not only to support certain diagnostic aspects but to demonstrate the unusual degree of self-deception practiced by the patient.

1. The MMPI record is valid in the sense that the respondent understood the items and responded consistently (TR + CLS = 0; ME = 51).

2. Patient is not seriously emotionally disturbed (XF+% = 84; P = 5; no qualitative indicators of an underlying thought process; PSY = T39; no scorable response on I-RD).

3. But she is nevertheless a chronically unhappy woman who is engaged in a massive denial of a number of unacceptable conditions. Hostility: OH = T68 and HOS = T38, Ho = T38, TSC/R = T35, that is, the respondent denies and represses hostile feelings. This interpretation is supported by 10% anatomy responses in the Rorschach content (i.e., bony anatomy = repressed hostility; Depression: DEP and TSC/D had raw scores of zero). Such remarkably low scores alone suggest denial. In addition, YF, a depression indicator, appeared among the Rorschach determinants, and D-S = T61—at least a trait depression is indicated. Dependency: I-Do = T51 and I-De = T29, a pair of scores that ordinarily suggests a self-assured person with low dependency needs. But three FY on the Rorschach is a clear dependency indicator, especially with two of them scored minus for response-quality—a sign of conflict in the area. Anxiety: TSC/T = T27 and PHO had no scorable responses, again the unusually low scores pointing to denial. Also, the presence of FY– in the Rorschach record suggests that anxiety accompanies conflict. Gender Identity: FEM = T42 and Astvn = T60, the combination appears to represent a woman who is not typically feminine. However, the Rorschach content was heavily feminine including such responses as women cooking or dancing, flowers, and fountains.

4. The patient perceives herself as moral, virtuous, and ingenuous (3NA = T69; 6N = T62; also E/Cy = 37 and 9AMO = 45). She claims to endorse basic American cultural values (5C = T75; L = T63).

5. She is comfortable with people, makes friends easily and enjoys social interaction (3DSA = T65; 4SI = T62 and 9IMP = T65; Rorschach Human % = 15; no depersonalized human responses; H greater than Hd).

The full report read as follows:

The patient is defensive in her general approach to mental investigation and makes extensive use of denial. She is not psychotic though it is likely that she is denying depression and anxiety.

The testing reveals several important conflicts. The patient has a very feminine aspect to her personality which is characterized by passive-dependency and a naive view of the world in which she perceives herself as moral, virtuous and stereotypically feminine. These characteristics are apparently making it difficult for the patient to maintain her managerial role in which males are both peers and subordinates. Thus, she denies her dependency needs and attempts to be hard, assertive and masculine. The intra-psychic struggle is further complicated by the fact that the patient has difficulty expressing hostility which she characteristically denies and represses.

The patient is socially comfortable and gregarious which, along with her inability to express hostility, serve her dependency needs well. However, since her comfort in relating socially is as a female, this aspect of the personality does not lend to her performance as a manager.

The patient's conflict has become so intense that she finds a temporary resolution by developing psychogenic physical complaints. Three years ago, an organic condition served the same purpose for her. Indeed, that experience may well have been the basis on which the current symptomatology was developed. In each case, the patient was incapacitated and unable to work for considerable periods of time, extricating herself temporarily from her identity-occupational conflict.

It appears that the patient is more comfortable as the stereotyped woman. Outpatient psychotherapy is recommended in which the therapist should explore the patient's occupational goals thoroughly.

The Case of SV

SV was a 38-year-old, white, married female, a college graduate, who was seen as an outpatient. On clinical examination, the patient appeared somewhat depressed but not nearly to a degree to account for the frequency of crying episodes. The patient's mood was dysphoric but she appeared to be functioning adequately.

The conjoint analysis follows:

1. The record is considered to be valid in that the patient's comprehension was adequate (TR + CLS = 3). However, the ME of 76 with four K-corrected clinical scales above T80 strongly indicates that this is a typical "cry for help" record in which the symptom picture is exaggerated.

2. The patient is very unhappy with her life space at the moment but she is not clinically depressed although DEP = T86 and TSC/D = T94. There are three morbid responses in the Rorschach content (all squashed animals) which contribute to the impression of some dysphoria. However, notably D-S = T50 and the Rorschach record contains six color responses including four that are FC+ and no achromatic color determination, all going counter to the presence of depression.

3. As usual, the exaggeration of symptoms is accomplished with anxiety and depression scales. The patient wants it to be known that she is very disturbed but not psychotic. Thus, I-RD = T45, I-DS = T48 and PSY = T55. The Rorschach picture actually seems a bit more disturbed with XF+% = 59 and $P = 4$, low for a response total of 27. Blood is found in two of the squashed animal responses and there is a third blood response that is Pure C. All told, there is enough to suggest that the patient is indeed beset by anxiety and depression though her exaggeration makes it difficult to determine the extent of either symptom.

4. The patient's personality has a marked obsessive-compulsive quality as evidenced by I-OC = T60 and Rorschach Dd% = 11. The latter is not as revealing as some of the patient's remarks during the administration, such as "I don't want to bias the inkblots by sex," "I'm concerned about doing this, to get the most out of it," "the drawing appears awkward," "I hate for this to be put down on paper," but "I want to be honest," "I panic when I can't think."

5. The patient has strong dependency needs (I-De = T70 and I-Do = 38; supporting Rorschach content includes a lamb, a smile, "little bugs," and "two hands reaching out").

6. The patient describes her family atmosphere as highly unpleasant (4FD = T80 and FAM = T66 despite the fact that the patient omitted five items that appear on one or the other of these scales).

7. The patient has a serious problem with gender identity and very likely with sexual behavior itself. The indicators of these three phenomena are salient in both test instruments. To begin with, FEM = T39 which is not all that indicative in a college-educated woman especially along with Astvn = T43. But I-SP = T97. The patient endorsed the item "Sexual things disgust me" and did not respond to the item "I am strongly attracted by members of my own sex." The patient gave six sex responses, an enormous number in a Rorschach record of any length. Furthermore, two of them were penises, a more psychopathological response because of its relative infrequency compared to female genitalia responses. The patient's Pure C response was "someone having a period." She remarked in the inquiry "I am not pleased at being a female." The patient perceived the popular female figures on Card VII. On Card VIII she began by saying "Every place where there's a fold—I can see this must be a drawing of female sexual—" and in the inquiry, she noted that she had seen female genitalia on Card VII as well but had suppressed the response. She remarked spontaneously that "It sounds gay to see two women and then a vulva."

8. The patient's family difficulties and her problems with gender identity have led her to feel isolated, different, misunderstood, and lacking a social support system (4SOA = T70; 8SOA = T84; Ho = T70). Hostility is typically expressed in resentment and irritability (TSC/R = T66); the patient has difficulty expressing aggression in a more mature fashion (HOS = T58).

The text of the complete report follows:

Most of the symptom picture is obtained from the MMPI which shows clear evidence of exaggeration. The symptom picture should, therefore, be viewed with extreme caution and is presented here only for purposes of completion of the report. The patient reports herself to be high anxiety-prone and chronically tense with multiple phobias. She feels extremely unhappy and guilt ridden but is not clinically depressed. A major problem appears to be cognitive retardation; the patient reports that her memory is poor and that she cannot concentrate or think logically and clearly. This deficit apparently occurs whenever the patient feels stressed. Crying appears to be a learned stress reaction and does not necessarily indicate dysphoric mood. Even the patient's occasional suicidal urge is more likely to have been motivated by obsessive–compulsive tendencies rather than by extreme depression. The patient also reports minor physical complaints of the type usually associated with emotional illness such as vague pains, easy fatigability, and general malaise. The patient has strong feelings of isolation, of being different and misunderstood and socially unsupported. These feelings are probably a consequence of frustration of strong dependency needs. The consequent hostility is expressed in an adolescent fashion by negativism and irritability since the patient has difficulty expressing hostility in a more adult fashion.

The patient is acutely unhappy with her family situation. She views the family milieu as quarrelsome, unpleasant, lacking in affection, overcontrolling, and infantilizing. It is most probable that these perceptions are attributable to her husband whom she blames for the frustration of her dependency needs. The patient's husband may have become alienated himself because the patient has a serious problem in gender identity which likely expresses itself in sexual behavior as well. She appears to reject heterosexual love and the stereotyped female role. She lacks many ordinary feminine interests and consciously wished that she were not a woman. Nevertheless, she appears preoccupied by sex. There is a good possibility of an underlying homosexual tendency of which the patient herself appears to have some awareness.

The Case of CI

The patient was an 18-year-old, single, white, outpatient male. He had contracted a minor illness which kept him from school for a week. After remission of symptoms, he had simply declined to leave his home and had not done so for a year and a half. He read and watched television and seemed totally unmotivated to do anything else despite various attempts at remediation by his parents. The referring psychiatrist requested information about the possibility of a schizoid personality or underlying thought disorder and the nature and extent of the patient's fantasy level.

The conjoint analysis follows:

1. The record was considered to be valid in that the patient comprehended the test items and responded truthfully to the best of his ability (TR + CLS = 2; ME = 59).

2. The patient is clearly not psychotic nor is there any evidence of an underlying thought disorder (I-RD = T46; PSY = T48; XF+% = 83; P = 5; no sex, anatomy, morbid, or blood responses and no qualitative indicators of thought disorder).

3. There is no evidence of either anxiety or depression (TSC/T = T40; PHO = T40; TSC/D = T45; DEP = T40; no YF and no content indicators).

4. There is some guilt present (the lone FC is minus).

5. The patient is heavily given to fantasy, not all of which is mature but none seems to be regressive or paranoid (six M+ and three AM responses, almost 70% of the response total; there are no paranoid indicators or ideation in the Rorschach and TSC/S = T37 with I-RD = T46).

6. The patient is a passive–dependent personality characterized by an acute lack of energy or need for stimulation (I-De = T75 and I-Do = T45; FY = 3 and there is a repeated use of the word "little" in the Rorschach record; 9PMA = T37, remarkably low for an 18-year-old male; HYP = T38 which lends support to the interpretation of passivity and adds a quality of stolidity to the personality picture).

7. The patient denies that he is socially uncomfortable (3DSA = T62; 4SI = T59; 9IMP = T49) and also denies that he tends to withdraw under stress (TSC/I = T41 and SOC = T43); the Rorschach supports the patient's perception of himself (H% = 31).

8. The patient has limited ability to express hostility and some tendency to deny and repress it (HOS = T45; AUT = T37; TSC/R = T41, all very low for an 18-year-old male; and OH = T55, suggestive although not definitive).

9. The patient has stereotypic feminine interests in the extreme (FEM = T65; feminine Rorschach content—music, botany, and dancing responses).

10. Not surprisingly, the patient acknowledges that he has a sex problem although he denies that it is homosexuality and it does not appear to be a paraphilia (I-SP = T74 but Pe = T46 and there are no diagnostic critical items; no sex content on the Rorschach suggests that the patient's sexual problem is conscious and not overwhelming).

11. The patient describes himself as moral and virtuous, specifically endorsing traditional national ideals with the exception of religion which is strongly and specifically rejected (6N = T61; 3NA = T64, both unusually high for an 18-year-old male; 5C = T70 but REL = T33).

12. Family problems are denied but there is some indication of difficulty with his mother (4FD = T48; FAM = T52 but the only female percept on the Rorschach is a witch, "devious, doing something, I can't tell what").

The text of the complete report follows:

The patient is not psychotic and there is no evidence of an underlying thought disorder or of paranoid or regressive ideation. The patient does not seem to have a problem either with anxiety or depression though he has some guilt feelings, probably related to hostility toward his mother.

The basic personality structure is passive-dependent and would probably be more appropriate for a female than a male. The life style and interests are typically feminine. The patient lacks conventional masculine ambitions and is somewhat naive and trusting in his interpersonal relationships. Despite his lack of ambition, he places a high value on traditional American ideals except for religion which is strongly rejected for some idiosyncratic reason.

The patient tends to deny hostility and his optimum stimulation level is low for an adolescent male; he is somewhat retarded psychomotorically.

The patient acknowledges that he has a sex problem but its specific nature is unclear. He denies that he is a homosexual despite the strong feminine interest pattern. There is no evidence that the patient has a paraphilia of any kind. This is an area which requires further exploration.

The patient, despite his withdrawal from the community, is probably socially comfortable though it is equally probable that he lacks sufficient motivation or drive to build a social support system. Certainly he could not be characterized as a schizoid personality.

The patient appears to have some resentment toward his mother though it is denied. The resentment may have sprung up recently, a reaction to the fact that his mother accepted his unconventional behavior for a long time but now sees him as in need of professional intervention.

A plausible hypothesis is that the patient's withdrawal from the community is a function of his recognition of his personality inversion. The purpose of the withdrawal is to escape rejection and ridicule.

CHAPTER 7
THE FATE OF ORIGINAL MMPI SPECIAL SCALES IN MMPI-2

Seventy items in the original MMPI underwent modification in MMPI-2 (Levitt, 1990).[14] According to Levitt's analysis, only four of these items have been altered substantially, and Ben-Porath and Butcher (1989) suggest that item modifications have little effect on responses.

Ninety items in MMPI-1 do not appear in MMPI-2 (Levitt, 1990). Since the special scales were all developed from the original MMPI, these deletions could have considerable impact on the scales' measurement viability when MMPI-2 is administered to a respondent. The developers of MMPI-2 (Butcher et al., 1989; Graham, 1990) evidently believe that the item deletions have seriously damaged the special scales and there is no indication that they intend to revive employment of the special scales by publishing new norms for them. The contention that the

---

[14]When the two existing versions of the MMPI are compared or otherwise mentioned in the same context, a need to differentiate between them arises. The restandardizers themselves employed the adjective, "original" to identify the earlier version (e.g., Butcher et al., 1989, pp. 1, 21, 107; Graham, 1990, pp. ix, 8, 15). This is the approach we have adopted in this book up to this point. The assessment community at large has gone in a different direction. The original MMPI is being referred to only as MMPI (e.g., Chojnacki & Walsh, 1994; Edwards, Morrison, & Weissman, 1993; Whitworth & McBlaine, 1993). Greene (1991) points out that this way of distinguishing "sometimes results in awkward referencing to the MMPI-2 or the MMPI within the same section" (p. ix). Nevertheless, Greene also adopts this distinction. Levitt and his coworkers solved the problem by calling the original version, MMPI-1. This neat differential is employed in this chapter because the exposition is based on articles in which it appears (Levitt, 1990; Levitt, Browning, & Freeland, 1992; Webb, Levitt, & Rodjdev, 1993).

special scales are no longer usable clinically can be subjected to empirical examination with considerable applied significance in view of a survey that indicates that MMPI-2 is slowly overtaking its predecessor in usage popularity, although a sizeable minority will remain loyal to the original form (Webb, Levitt, & Rojdev, 1993). A significant question emerges from these observations: To what extent can the clinician who administers MMPI-2 still make use of the special scales?

In an effort to formulate a reply, Levitt (1990) performed a structural analysis of the impact on MMPI-1 special scales that result from the changes made in MMPI-2. He found that effects on the Harris and Lingoes (1968) scales were minimal, not at all surprising since the MMPI clinical scales themselves were also minimally affected by item loss. All subscales remain as they were in the original Harris and Lingoes content partitioning, except for the changes reflected in Table 7.1. Twenty-two of the 28 subscales are unchanged. All of the subscales that remain intact are omitted from Table 7.1; only those subscales appear that were diminished by item deletion.

Harris and Lingoes Psychomotor Retardation subscale (2PR) lost only a single item. All five subscales that were derived from Scale 4 were reduced in length, again not surprising in view of the items added to these subscales by Harris and Lingoes.[15] These losses were considerable, ranging from 18.2% for Familial Discord (4FD) to 50.0% for Social Imperturbability (4SI). For the six affected subscales, a total of 20 items were lost, an average of 3.3 items per subscale. Considering all Harris and Lingoes subscales, including those unaffected by the MMPI-2 revision, the loss per subscale is only 0.7 items.

Among the 13 Wiggins (1966) content scales, 10 shrank in length as a result of the revision but only Religious Fundamentalism (REL) was thoroughly decimated (Table 7.1). Aside from REL, for the remaining nine altered scales the item loss percent ranged from a low of 3.7% for Social Maladjustment (SOC) and Phobias (PHO) to a high of 32.1% for Poor Health (HEA). From the perspective of numbers of items lost, a total of 41 scored on the Wiggins scales became unavailable for use in MMPI-2. This amounts to an average of 4.1 items per scale for affected scales. Omitting REL, the average loss is 3.3 items per scale; for the affected plus intact scales, 2.5 items per scale.

The precise effect of item loss is impossible to gauge accurately from structural analysis. However, for the majority of these scales, it may well be inconsequential. Wiggins' own pessimistic view that his quarter-of-a-century-old scales are dead (Wiggins, 1990) may be premature. The Wiggins scales may, in fact, turn out to be hardier than either the MMPI-2 revision team (Butcher et al., 1989) or their creator believes. The continuing potential of these scales is strongly suggested by the relationships and reliabilities that are reviewed in Table 8.4 of this book.

---

[15]Harris and Lingoes (1955) included 14 items that were allegedly found in an early version of Scale 4 but do not appear in the published form.

TABLE 7.1
MMPI-1 Special Scales Shortened by MMPI-2 Revision[1]

Special Scale[2]		Number of Items		
		MMPI-1	MMPI-2	% Items Lost
Harris-Lingoes Subscales				
2PR	(Psychomotor Retardation)	15	14	6.7
4FD	(Familial Discord)	11	9	18.2
4AC	(Authority Conflict)	11	8	27.3
4SI	(Social Imperturbability)	12	6	50.0
4SOA	(Social Alienation)	18	13	27.8
4SEA	(Self-Alienation)	15	12	20.0
Wiggins Content Scales				
SOC	(Social Maladjustment)	27	26	3.7
FEM	(Feminine Interests)	30	23	23.3
REL	(Religious Fundamentalism)	12	1	91.7
MOR	(Poor Morale)	23	22	4.3
PSY	(Psychoticism)	48	45	6.2
ORG	(Organic Symptoms)	36	32	11.1
HOS	(Manifest Hostility	27	25	7.4
PHO	(Phobias)	27	26	3.7
HYP	(Hypomania)	25	23	8.0
HEA	(Poor Health)	28	19	32.1
Tryon, Stein, and Chu Cluster Scales				
TSC/A	(Autism)	23	20	13.0
TSC/B	(Body Symptoms)	33	32	3.0
TSC/I	(Social Introversion)	26	25	3.8
TSC/T	(Tension)	35	34	2.9
Indiana Rational Scales				
I-DS	(Dissociative Symptoms)	8	7	12.5
I-Do	(Dominance)	17	15	11.8
I-RD	(Severe Reality Distortion)	16	15	6.2
I-SP	(Sex Problems-Female)	12	8	33.3
I-SP	(Sex Problems-Male)	14	9	35.7
Other Scales				
AMac	(Alcoholism, MacAndrew)	51	46	9.8
CLS	(Carelessness)	12	10	16.7
Cn	(Control)	49	43	12.2
E/Cy	(Cynicism-Female)	20	19	5.0
E/Cy	(Cynicism-Male)	20	18	10.0
OH	(Overcontrolled Hostility)	31	28	9.7
Pe	(Pedophilia)	24	20	16.7
WA	(Work Attitude)	37	36	2.7

[1]MMPI-1 special scales not altered in MMPI-2 are omitted from Table 7.1.
[2]Sources of special scales are all cited in text.

Three of the seven Tryon, Stein, and Chu scales (Stein, 1968), TSC/D, TSC/R, TSC/S, were unaffected by the revision. Only small numbers of items were lost from the remaining four scales (Table 7.1). The Autism scale (TSC/A), which Levitt (1989) did not find to be clinically useful, was most affected, with a loss of 13.0% of its items. The remaining three scales each lost less than 4% of its items. Overall, only six items were lost, an average of 1.5 items per affected scale. Considering all seven Tryon, Stein, and Chu scales, this average drops to 0.9 items per scale.

Analysis of the seven Indiana Rational scales (Levitt, 1989) revealed that three were unaffected. The Sex Problems scale (I-SP), was most affected, with losses of 33.3% of items for females to 35.7% for males (Table 7.1). The remaining three affected Indiana scales lost between 6.2% and 12.5% of their items. Using the average items lost for the male and female versions of I-SP, a total of 8.5 items was lost from four scales, for an average item loss per scale of 2.1. Adding to this the three unaffected Indiana scales, the average item loss drops to 1.2 per scale.

For the 10 additional special scales, which were drawn from a variety of sources (see review pp. 41–46), three were unchanged by the MMPI-2 revision: Conventionality (5C) (Pepper & Strong, 1958; Levitt, 1989), Extreme Suspiciousness (S+) (Endicott, Jortner, & Abramoff, 1969), and Hostility (Ho) (Cook & Medley, 1954). The items available for scoring Cynicism (E/Cy) (Eichman, 1961 for females; Eichman, 1962 for males) dropped slightly for both the male and female versions of the scale (5.0% for females and 10.0% for males) (Table 7.1). Alterations for the six remaining special scales ranged from under 3% for Work Attitude (WA) (Tydlaska & Mengel, 1953) to 16.7% for Carelessness (CLS) (Greene, 1978) and Pedophilia (Pe) (Toobert, Bartelme, & Jones, 1959). Other affected scales are: Alcoholism (AMac) (MacAndrew, 1965)—9.8%; Control (Cn) (Cuadra, 1956)—12.2%; and Overcontrolled Hostility (OH) (Megargee, Cook, & Mendelsohn, 1967)—9.7%.

If the item loss for E/Cy is used across the female and male scorings, the total average item loss for affected scales from the "Other Scales" in Table 7.1, is 22.5. For the seven affected scales this results in an average loss of 3.2 items per scale. Including with these the three scales unaffected by the revision, the average loss becomes 2.2 items per scale. Subject to further empirical study, all of these special scales including the E/Cy's appear still to be usable.

An overall conclusion can be drawn from Levitt's (1990) structural analysis of the MMPI-1 special scales. Due to the preservation in MMPI-2 of 83.6% of the MMPI-1 items either in their original or slightly modified form, most of the MMPI-1 special scales remain intact or have undergone only limited item loss. Specifically, of the total group of 65 different special scales considered, 34 or 52.3% are unchanged. Of the remaining 31 special scales that lost items in MMPI-2, the average loss per scale is 17.6%. If one omits from this calculation the two scales whose item losses were 50.0% or more (REL and 4SI are essentially

TABLE 7.2
Magnitude of Absolute Differences Between Special Scale Means
From MMPI-1 and MMPI-2 Items

	Psychiatric Sample		Normal Sample		Total Sample	
Difference	Frequency	%	Frequency	%	Frequency	%
≥ 3.0	3	5.3	3	5.3	6	5.3
2.0–2.99	6	10.5	2	3.5	8	7.0
1.0–1.99	16	28.1	10	17.5	26	22.8
.50–.99	16	28.1	17	29.3	33	28.9
< .5	16	28.1	25	43.9	41	36.0
Total < 1.0	32	56.1	42	73.7	74	64.9
Total	57	100.0	57	100.0	114	100.0

Note. Data derived from comparisons of 29 scales for male samples and 28 scales for female samples (Pedophilia scale is not scored for females) (Table 6 in Levitt et al., 1992, p. 28).

lost scales), the loss for 29 special scales is just under 14%. The next step is a more precise empirical evaluation of how well the altered special scales have retained their measurement utility.

EMPIRICAL COMPARABILITY
OF REVISED SPECIAL SCALES

Levitt, Browning, and Freeland (1992) undertook a study to clarify how much special scale mean scores might be changed by the loss of items in MMPI-2. All of the altered special scales listed in Table 7.1 were included with the exception of REL and 2PR.[16]

Samples of normals' and psychiatric inpatients' MMPI-1 records were scored in the standard manner for the altered special scales. Scales were scored a second time, omitting those items deleted in the MMPI-2 revision. Comparisons were made between the obtained raw score means from the two scoring procedures. Within the normal sample, 73.7% of the scale means differed less than one raw score point across the pool of 29 special scales examined (Table 7.2, which is Table 6 in Levitt et al., 1992). Due to the fact that overall larger scores were obtained by the psychiatric inpatients, fewer of their special scale means— 56.1%—differed by one raw score point or less. Nevertheless, only 5.3% of the scale means differed by as much as three or more raw score points for either normals or for psychiatric inpatients (Table 7.2).

---

[16]2PR was inadvertently omitted from the analyses carried out by Levitt et al. (1992). We note that the overall mean difference for 2PR for the psychiatric sample is 0.72, for the normal sample, 0.70. Evidently, the inclusion of these data would have no noticeable effect on the data in Tables 7.2 and 7.3.

TABLE 7.3

Median Scores of the Distributions of Differences Between Special Scale Means
Scored From MMPI-1 and MMPI-2 Items

Scale Groups	Psychiatric Sample Median	Normal Sample Median
Harris-Lingoes	1.69	.03
Wiggins	.64	.605
Tryon, Stein, & Chu	.44	.335
Indiana Rational	.55	.40
Other	1.48	1.60

Note.   Based on Table 7 (Levitt et al., 1992, p. 29).

Another perspective on the effect of item losses is obtained by a reframing of the data in Table 7.2. The distributions of mean differences between MMPI-1 and MMPI-2 scores in Table 7.2 was determined for both genders for each of the five special scale groupings. The medians of these distributions of differences are shown in Table 7.3 which is adapted from Table 7 in Levitt et al. (1992). These medians more accurately portray the effect of item loss on the scoring of special scales. This effect appears to be minimal. The range of median differences for the normal sample is 0.03 to 1.60; only one median is greater than 0.61. The range for the psychiatric sample was 0.44 to 1.69; three of the five medians are less than 0.65. Levitt et al. (1992) conclude from their findings that

> ... most of the scales we examined are probably subject to the same interpretation when scored from MMPI-1 and MMPI-2 items. The Harris and Lingoes subscales of Scale 4; the Wiggins Feminine Interests, Organic Symptoms, Poor Health, and Religious Fundamentalism scales; the Control scale, and possibly the McAndrew Alcoholism scale are exceptions to this hypothesis. (p. 29)

As we have already noted, more than half of the special scales described in this book have passed into MMPI-2 unchanged except for some minor improvements in wording. With a few exceptions, among those scales that are shortened in MMPI-2, between one-third and one-half yielded mean scores that differed by one item point or less compared to the unshortened version. Summing these two findings, we may reasonably conclude that around 80% of the special scales discussed in this book can be interpreted from an MMPI-2 record using the data in Appendices III, IV, and VI.

CHAPTER 8
THE MMPI-2
CONTENT SCALES

The original MMPI clinical scales are essentially intact in the new version, MMPI-2. They inherit the shortcomings of the clinical scales noted in Chapter 1. As of early 1994, the only special scales for the measurement of personality and psychopathology that have been developed from the MMPI-2 item pool is a series of 15 content scales (Butcher, et al., 1989). The MMPI-2 Content scales are presented in this volume because of their striking resemblance to the useful Wiggins Content scales discussed in Chapter 3. The resemblance hints at the possibility that the MMPI-2 scales may also be found useful eventually.

The two sets of content scales share a common development methodology and have a substantial item overlap. Greene (1991) suggests that ten MMPI-2 scales are related by title to a specific Wiggins scale. According to Greene's computations, the range of item overlap among these pairs of scales is from 25% (Low Self-Esteem and Poor Morale) to 83% (Fears and Phobias; Bizarre Mentation and Psychoticism). The mean item overlap computed from Greene's data is 53.5%. In terms of correlation, *every* MMPI-2 scale has a clear counterpart among the Wiggins scales. This fact is clearly shown in Table 8.1. The data in the table are based on the MMPI-2 standardization sample (Butcher, Graham, Williams, & Ben-Porath, 1990).

All of the coefficients except one in Table 8.1 are at least .70 and more than half are higher than .80. Obviously, this correspondence is due in good part to the substantial item overlap. However, other factors also play an important role as illustrated by a rank-order correlation of only .53 between the item overlap

TABLE 8.1
The Relationship Between MMPI-2 Content Scales and
Selected Wiggins Content Scales

Reliability of MMPI-2 Content Scales		MMPI-2 Content Scales
T-R[a]	Alpha[b]	Correlations with Wiggins Content Scales
.87/.90	.83/.82	Anxiety [DEP .83/.80] [MOR .77/.74]
.86/.81	.75/.72	Fears [PHO .92/.91]
.85/.83	.77/.74	Obsessiveness [DEP .75/.69] [MOR .79/.72]
.85/.87	.86/.85	Depression [DEP .91/.89] [MOR .80/.79]
.85/.81	.80/.76	Health Concerns [ORG .84/.82] [HEA .81/.79]
.81/.78	.74/.73	Bizarre Mentation [PSY .82/.84]
.82/.85	.73/.76	Anger [HOS .80/.79]
.89/.80	.85/.86	Cynicism [AUT .87/.84]
.87/.81	.75/.78	Antisocial Practices [AUT .87/.88]
.79/.82	.68/.72	Type A Behavior [HOS .78/.80]
.86/.84	.83/.79	Low Self-Esteem [DEP .73/.70] [MOR .83/.79]
.90/.91	.84/.83	Social Discomfort [SOC .92/.92]
.83/.84	.77/.73	Family Problem [FAM .86/.82]
.91/.90	.84/.82	Work Interference [DEP .82/.79] [MOR .85/.82]
.88/.79	.80/.78	Negative Treatment Indicators [DEP .76/.75] [MOR .78/.75]

Note. Data from Butcher et al. (1990). Female sample before slash, male after it.
[a]Test-retest.
[b]Cronbach's (1951) coefficient.

in the scales analyzed by Greene (1991) and the respective gender-averaged correlation coefficient in Table 8.1.

The reliabilities of the MMPI-2 scales are also presented in Table 8.1 for contrast. It can readily be seen that the MMPI-2 scales–Wiggins scales intercorrelations compare favorably with the reliabilities of the MMPI-2 scales. In fact, the scale intercorrelations are generally higher than the Cronbach alphas, a stronger measure of reliability than the test-retest coefficients. The alphas are based on the total normative sample—at least a thousand cases—while the test-retest coefficients were derived from only 111 female subjects and 82 males.

Thus far, the correlations with the well-established Wiggins scales are the best evidence of validity for the MMPI-2 scales. Several other efforts to demonstrate validity are described by Butcher, Graham, Williams, and Ben-Porath (1990). Eight-hundred and twenty-two subjects in the MMPI-2 standardization sample, most of them married, rated each other on a series of personality, behavior and symptom statements. Among the statistically significant correlations between various statements and MMPI-2 scales few reached as high as .30. The MMPI-2 Work Interference scale (WRK) differentiated among samples of airplane pilots, military personnel, alcoholics and other psychiatric patients in the theoretically anticipated direction. However, any number of construct measures might have done as well; thus, the validity demonstration for WRK is weak. The Health

Concerns scale (HEA) sharply differentiated chronic pain patients from normals, as would be expected by any measure of admission of physical symptoms. Psychiatric patients scored higher than the pain sufferers on all MMPI-2 content scales except HEA including scales for the measurement of anxiety, depression and bizarre thinking.

A few other reports also may bear on the validity of MMPI-2 Content scales. Schill and Wang (1990) found that the Anger scale correlated significantly with five of 11 other anger measures in female subjects and seven of 11 in male subjects. Several content scales helped to differentiate schizophrenics from patients suffering from a major depression (Ben-Porath, Butcher, & Graham, 1991). An investigation by Ben-Porath, McCully, and Almagor (1993) suggests that the content scales may be more effective measures of psychopathology and some personality characteristics than the MMPI-2 clinical scales. Butcher (1994) reports content scale data on a sample of 437 applicants for jobs as airline pilots. Not unexpectedly, significant defensiveness is apparent on all content scales with the applicants averaging more than 10 T-score points below the MMPI-2 male normative sample. On the way to a well-designed demonstration that various Rorschach indices (Exner, 1993) are valid only when the response total is around 30, Meyer (1993) found positive correlations between some Rorschach indices and appropriate MMPI-2 Content scales in a subsample with a high response total. For example, the Rorschach Depression Index had strong positive correlations with the Depression, Low-Self Esteem and Work Interference content scales. The Rorschach Obsessive Style Index was related to the Anxiety and Depression content scales (but not to the Obsessiveness content scale). However, Bizarre Mentation, Cynicism and Fears contents scales were unrelated to the Rorschach Hypervigilance Index.

The developers of the MMPI-2 Content scales believe that the available validity data are "an encouraging first look" but "further studies will be necessary to obtain a clearer and more detailed picture of their usefulness in clinical assessment" (Butcher et al., 1990, p. 95). Graham (1990) also comments that "the preliminary data ... is impressive and encouraging" but "more empirical data are needed before the validity of the content scales can be judged adequately" (p. 131).

In light of the marked relationship between MMPI-2 and Wiggins Content scales, the eventual contribution of the former may be limited, despite "the encouraging first look." At this time, the Wiggins Content scales continue to be clinically useful, even when scored from an MMPI-2 record. The MMPI-2 Content scales may eventually catch up with or even overtake their antecedent scales but this remains to be demonstrated by considerable future research.

APPENDIX I
SPECIAL SCALES:
ITEM COMPOSITION
AND SOURCES

Wiggins Content Scales*

SOC—Social Maladjustment
  True: 52, 171, 172, 180, 201, 267, 292, 304, 377, 384, 453, 455, 509
  False: 57, 91, 99, 309, 371, 391, 449, 450, 479, 482, 502, 520, 521, 547
DEP—Depression
  True: 41, 61, 67, 76, 94, 104, 106, 158, 202, 209, 210, 217, 259, 305, 337, 338, 339, 374, 390, 396, 413, 414, 487, 517, 518, 526, 543
  False: 8, 79, 88, 207, 379, 407
FEM Feminine Interests
  True: 70, 74, 77, 78, 87, 92, 126, 132, 140, 149, 203, 261, 295, 463, 538, 554, 557, 562
  False: 1, 81, 219, 221, 223, 283, 300, 423, 434, 537, 552, 563

---

*Source: Wiggins, 1966. (Copyright 1966 by the American Psychological Association. Reprinted by permission.)

MOR—Poor Morale
  True: 84, 86, 138, 142, 244, 321, 357, 361, 375, 382, 389, 395, 397, 398, 411, 416, 418, 431, 531, 549, 555
  False: 122, 264
REL—Religious Fundamentalism
  True: 58, 95, 98, 115, 206, 249, 258, 373, 483, 488, 490
  False: 491
AUT—Authority Conflict
  True: 59, 71, 93, 116, 117, 118, 124, 250, 265, 277, 280, 298, 313, 316, 319, 406, 436, 437, 446
  False: 294
PSY—Psychoticism
  True: 16, 22, 24, 27, 33, 35, 40, 48, 50, 66, 73, 110, 121, 123, 127, 136, 151, 168, 184, 194, 197, 200, 232, 275, 278, 284, 291, 293, 299, 312, 317, 334, 341, 345, 348, 349, 350, 364, 400, 420, 433, 448, 476, 511, 551
  False: 198, 347, 464

111

ORG—Organic Symptoms

True: 23, 44, 108, 114, 156, 159, 161, 186, 189, 251, 273, 332, 335, 541, 560

False: 46, 68, 103, 119, 154, 174, 175, 178, 185, 187, 188, 190, 192, 243, 274, 281, 330, 405, 496, 508, 540

FAM—Family Problems

True: 21, 212, 216, 224, 226, 239, 245, 325, 327, 421, 516

False: 65, 96, 137, 220, 527

HOS—Manifest Hostility

True: 28, 39, 80, 89, 109, 129, 139, 145, 162, 218, 269, 282, 336, 355, 363, 368, 393, 410, 417, 426, 438, 447, 452, 468, 469, 495, 536

False: None

PHO—Phobias

True: 166, 182, 351, 352, 360, 365, 385, 388, 392, 473, 480, 492, 494, 499, 525, 553

False: 128, 131, 169, 176, 287, 353, 367, 401, 412, 522, 539

HYP—Hypomania

True: 13, 134, 146, 181, 196, 228, 234, 238, 248, 266, 268, 272, 296, 340, 342, 372, 381, 386, 409, 439, 445, 465, 500, 505, 506

False: None

HEA—Poor Health

True: 10, 14, 29, 34, 72, 125, 279, 424, 519, 544

False: 2, 18, 36, 51, 55, 63, 130, 153, 155, 163, 193, 214, 230, 462, 474, 486, 533, 542

False: 57, 79, 264, 309, 353, 371, 415, 449, 479, 482, 521, 547

TSC/B—Body Symptoms

True: 10, 14, 23, 29, 44, 47, 62, 72, 108, 114, 125, 161, 189, 191, 263, 544

False: 2, 3, 18, 36, 51, 55, 68, 103, 153, 160, 163, 175, 190, 192, 230, 243, 330

TSC/S—Suspicion

True: 71, 89, 112, 136, 244, 265, 278, 280, 284, 316, 319, 348, 368, 383, 390, 404, 406, 426, 436, 438, 447, 455, 469, 507, 558

False: None

TSC/D—Depression

True: 41, 61, 67, 76, 84, 104, 142, 168, 236, 259, 301, 339, 357, 361, 384, 396, 397, 411, 414, 418, 487, 526, 549

False: 8, 46, 88, 107, 379

TSC/R—Resentment

True: 28, 39, 94, 97, 106, 129, 139, 145, 147, 148, 162, 234, 336, 375, 381, 382, 416, 443, 468, 536

False: None

TSC/T—Tension

True: 13, 22, 32, 43, 102, 158, 166, 182, 186, 217, 238, 303, 322, 335, 337, 338, 340, 351, 360, 365, 388, 431, 439, 442, 448, 473, 492, 494, 499, 506, 543, 555

False: 131, 152, 242, 407

Composition of Tryon, Stein, and Chu Cluster Scales*

TSC/I—Social Introversion

True: 52, 86, 138, 171, 172, 180, 201, 267, 292, 304, 317, 321, 377, 509

Composition of Indiana Rational Scales

I-De—Dependency Inventory

True: 141, 143, 165, 394, 398, 531, 564

False: 170, 235, 501

*Source: Stein, 1968. (Reprinted with permission of the author.)

I-DS—Dissociative Symptoms Inventory
  True: 22, 50, 156, 194, 251, 345, 420
  False: 464
I-Do—Dominance Inventory
  True: 79, 112, 170, 235, 257, 264, 404,
    415, 426, 432, 447, 502, 520
  False: 82, 444, 503, 509
I-OC—Obsessive-Compulsiveness Inventory
  True: 64, 213, 343, 346, 358, 359,
    414, 461, 467
  False: None
I-SC—Self-Concept Inventory
  True: 74 (for males), 84, 86, 106,
    142, 209, 418, 517
  False: 54, 73, 74 (for females), 122,
    257, 262, 264
I-RD—Severe Reality Distortion Inventory
  True: 27, 33, 48, 50, 66, 121, 123,
    151, 184, 200, 275, 291, 334,
    345, 349, 350, 476
  False: 464
I-SP—Sex Problems Inventory
  True: 69, 74 (for males), 85, 179,
    297, 320, 470, 519, 548 (for
    males), 558 (for males)
  False: 20, 37, 74 (for females), 133,
    430

Composition of Harris & Lingoes Scales

Scale 2—Depression

D_1—Subjective Depression = 2SD
  True: 32, 41, 43, 52, 67, 86, 104,
    138, 142, 158, 159, 182, 189,
    236, 259
  False: 2, 8, 46, 57, 88, 107, 122, 131,
    152, 160, 191, 207, 208, 242,
    272, 285, 296
D_2—Psychomotor Retardation = 2PR
  True: 41, 52, 182, 259
  False: 8, 30, 39, 57, 64, 89, 95, 145,
    207, 208, 233

D_3—Physical Malfunctioning = 2PM
  True: 130, 189, 193, 288
  False: 2, 18, 51, 153, 154, 155, 160
D_4—Mental Dullness = 2MD
  True: 32, 41, 86, 104, 159, 182, 259,
    290
  False: 8, 9, 46, 88, 122, 178, 207

Scale 3—Hysteria

Hy_1—Denial of Society Anxiety = 3DSA
  True: None
  False: 141, 172, 180, 201, 267, 292
Hy_2—Need for Affection = 3NA
  True: 253
  False: 26, 71, 89, 93, 109, 124, 136,
    162, 234, 265, 289
Hy_3—Lassitude-Malaise = 3LM
  True: 32, 43, 76, 189, 238
  False: 2, 3, 8, 9, 51, 107, 137, 153,
    160, 163
Hy_4—Somatic Complaints = 3SC
  True: 10, 23, 44, 47, 114, 186
  False: 7, 55, 103, 174, 175, 188, 190,
    192, 230, 243, 274

Scale 4—Psychopathic Deviate

Pd_1—Familial Discord = 4FD
  True: 21, 42, 212, 216, 224, 245
  False: 96, 137, 235, 237, 527
Pd_2—Authority Conflict = 4AC
  True: 38, 59, 118, 520
  False: 37, 82, 141, 173, 289, 294, 429
Pd_3—Social Imperturbability = 4SI
  True: 64, 479, 520, 521
  False: 82, 141, 171, 180, 201, 267,
    304, 352
Pd_{4A}—Social Alienation = 4SOA
  True: 16, 24, 35, 64, 67, 94, 110,
    127, 146, 239, 244, 284, 305,
    368, 520
  False: 20, 141, 170

Scale 6—Paranoia

Pa₁—Persecutory Ideas = 6PI
  True: 16, 24, 35, 110, 121, 123, 127,
    151, 157, 202, 275, 284, 291,
    293, 338, 364
  False: 347
Pa₂—Poignancy = 6P
  True: 24, 158, 299, 305, 317, 341, 365
  False: 111, 268
Pa₃—Naiveté = 6N
  True: 314
  False: 93, 109, 117, 124, 313, 316,
    319, 348

Scale 8—Schizophrenia

Sc₁ₐ—Social Alienation = 8SOA
  True: 16, 21, 24, 35, 52, 121, 157,
    212, 241, 282, 305, 312, 324,
    325, 352, 364
  False: 65, 220, 276, 306, 309
Sc₂ₐ—Lack of Ego Mastery, Cognitive =
8COG
  True: 32, 33, 159, 168, 182, 335, 345,
    349, 356
  False: 178
Sc₂ʙ—Lack of Ego Mastery, Conative =
8CON
  True: 32, 40, 41, 76, 104, 202, 259,
    301, 335, 339, 356
  False: 8, 196, 322
Sc₃—Bizarre Sensory Experiences = 8BSE
  True: 22, 33, 47, 156, 194, 210, 251,
    273, 291, 332, 334, 341, 345,
    350
  False: 103, 119, 187, 192, 281, 330

Scale 9—Hypomania

Ma₁—Amorality = 9AMO
  True: 143, 250, 271, 277, 298
  False: 289

Ma₂—Psychomotor Acceleration = 9PMA
  True: 13, 97, 100, 134, 181, 228, 238,
    266, 268
  False: 111, 119
Ma₃—Imperturbability = 9IMP
  True: 167, 222, 240
  False: 105, 148, 171, 180, 267

Other Scales

Astvn—Assertiveness (Female)
  True: 3, 28, 37, 45, 52, 54, 63, 101,
    122, 137, 163, 172, 178, 269,
    338, 344, 379, 383, 406, 415,
    432, 436, 458, 462, 474, 476,
    478, 481, 508, 513, 561, 562
  False: 22, 58, 64, 95, 98, 99, 158,
    209, 254, 276, 320, 326, 370, 394,
    459, 463, 464, 468, 525, 544, 554,
    557
5C—Conventionality
  True: None
  False: 19, 26, 28, 80, 89, 112, 117,
    120, 280
L—Lie Scale
  True: None
  False: 15, 30, 45, 60, 75, 90, 105,
    120, 135, 150, 165, 195, 225,
    255, 285
AMac: Alcoholism
  True: 6, 27, 34, 50, 56, 57, 58, 61, 81,
    94, 116, 118, 127, 128, 140, 156,
    186, 215, 224, 235, 243, 251, 263,
    283, 309, 413, 419, 426, 445, 446,
    477, 482, 483, 488, 500, 507, 529,
    562
  False: 86, 120, 130, 149, 173, 179, 278,
    294, 320, 335, 356, 378, 460
Cn: Control
  True: 6, 20, 30, 56, 67, 105, 116,
    134, 145, 162, 169, 181, 225,
    236, 238, 285, 296, 319, 337,
    382, 411, 418, 436, 446, 447,
    460, 529, 555

False: 58, 80, 92, 96, 111, 167, 174,
220, 242, 249, 250, 291, 313,
360, 378, 439, 444, 483, 488,
489, 527, 548

E/Cy: Cynicism (males)

True: 11, 28, 35, 89, 117, 157, 206,
213, 256, 265, 280, 286, 316,
319, 365, 454, 456

False: 54, 111, 347

E/Cy: Cynicism (females)

True: 11, 35, 89, 117, 183, 209, 213,
218, 245, 265, 280, 316, 319, 454,
465

False: 54, 111, 115, 306, 347

D-S: Depression, subtle

True: 5, 130, 193

False: 30, 39, 58, 64, 80, 89, 98, 145,
155, 160, 191, 208, 233, 241,
248, 263, 296

Ho: Hostility

True: 19, 28, 52, 59, 71, 89, 93, 110,
117, 124, 136, 148, 157, 183,
226, 244, 250, 252, 265, 271,
278, 280, 284, 292, 319, 348,
368, 383, 386, 394, 406, 410,
411, 426, 436, 438, 447, 455,
458, 469, 485, 504, 507, 520,
531, 551, 558

False: 237, 253, 399

CLS: Carelessness

Item Pair	Deviant Response
10–405	Same
17– 65	Different
18– 63	Different
49–113	Same
76–107	Same
88–526	Same
137–216	Same
177–220	Different
178–342	Same
286–312	Different
329–425	Same
388–480	Different

TR: Test-Retest

Item Pair
8–318
13–290
15–314
16–315
20–310
21–308
22–326
23–288
24–333
32–328
33–323
35–331
37–302
38–311
305–366
317–362

OH: Overcontrolled Hostility

True: 78, 91, 229, 319, 338, 373, 394,
425, 488, 559

False: 1, 30, 81, 90, 102, 109, 129,
130, 141, 165, 181, 183, 290,
329, 382, 396, 439, 446, 475,
501, 534

Pe: Pedophilia

True: 16, 53, 67, 76, 95, 106, 132,
179, 202, 206, 219, 260, 332,
390, 458, 490

False: 20, 57, 133, 160, 248, 276, 435,
556

S+: Extreme Suspiciousness

True: 27, 35, 110, 121, 123, 136, 151,
200, 265, 275, 278, 284, 291,
293, 348, 364, 384, 448

False: None

WA: Work Attitude

True: 13, 16, 32, 35, 40, 41, 59, 84,
109, 112, 170, 244, 250, 259,
272, 301, 312, 331, 335, 343,
389, 395, 404, 406, 435, 487,
507, 526, 549

False: 3, 9, 88, 164, 207, 257, 318, 407

Scale Title	Acronym	Source
Alcoholism	AMac	MacAndrew (1965)
Amorality	9AMO	Harris & Lingoes (1955)
Assertiveness	Astvn	Ohlson & Wilson (1974)
Authority Conflict	4AC	Harris & Lingoes (1955)
Authority Conflict	AUT	Wiggins (1966)
Bizarre Sensory Experiences	8BSE	Harris & Lingoes (1955)
Body Symptoms	TSC/B	Stein (1968)
Carelessness	CLS	Green (1978)
Conventionality	5C	Pepper & Strong (1958)
Control	Cn	Cuadra (1956)
Cynicism	E/Cy	Eichman (1961, 1962)
Denial of Social Anxiety	3DSA	Harris & Lingoes (1955)
Dependency	I-De	Levitt (1989)
Depression	DEP	Wiggins (1966)
Depression	TSC/D	Stein (1968)
Depression-Subtle	D-S	Wiener & Harmon (1946)
Dissociative Symptoms	I-DS	Levitt (1989)
Dominance	I-Do	Levitt (1989)
Extreme Suspiciousness	S+	Endicott et al. (1969)
Family Problems	FAM	Wiggins (1966)
Familial Discord	4FD	Harris & Lingoes (1955)
Feminine Interests	FEM	Wiggins (1966)
Hostility	Ho	Cook & Medley (1954)
Hypomania	HYP	Wiggins (1966)
Imperturbability	9IMP	Harris & Lingoes (1955)
Lack of Ego-Mastery, Cognitive	8COG	Harris & Lingoes (1955)
Lack of Ego-Mastery, Conative	8CON	Harris & Lingoes (1955)
Lie	L	Dahlstrom et al. (1972)
Manifest Hostility	HOS	Wiggins (1966)
Mean Elevation	ME	Modlin (1947)
Mental Dullness	2MD	Harris & Lingoes (1955)
Naiveté	6N	Harris & Lingoes (1955)
Need for Affection	3NA	Harris & Lingoes (1955)
Obsessive-Compulsiveness	I-OC	Levitt (1989)
Organic Symptoms	ORG	Wiggins (1966)
Overcontrolled Hostility	OH	Megargee et al. (1967)
Pedophilia	Pe	Toobert et al. (1959)
Phobias	PHO	Wiggins (1966)
Poignancy	6P	Harris & Lingoes (1955)
Poor Health	HEA	Wiggins (1966)
Poor Morale	MOR	Wiggins (1966)
Psychomotor Acceleration	9PMA	Harris & Lingoes (1955)
Psychomotor Retardation	2PR	Harris & Lingoes (1955)
Psychoticism	PSY	Wiggins (1966)
Religious Fundamentalism	REL	Wiggins (1966)
Resentment	TSC/R	Stein (1968)
Self-Concept	I-SC	Levitt (1989)

(Continued)

SOURCES
(Continued)

Scale Title	Acronym	Source
Severe Reality Distortions	I-RD	Levitt (1989)
Sex Problems	I-SP	Levitt (1989)
Social Alienation	4SOA	Harris & Lingoes (1955)
Social Alienation	8SOA	Harris & Lingoes (1955)
Social Imperturbability	4SI	Harris & Lingoes (1955)
Social Introversion	TSC/I	Stein (1968)
Social Maladjustment	SOC	Wiggins (1966)
Subjective Depression	2SD	Harris & Lingoes (1955)
Suspicion	TSC/S	Stein (1968)
Tension	TSC/T	Stein (1968)
Test-Retest	TR	Buechley & Ball (1952)
Work Attitude	WA	Tydlaska & Mengel (1953)

APPENDIX II
DEMOGRAPHIC DESCRIPTION
OF THE INDIANA SAMPLE*
(PERCENTS)

	Male	Female	% Total
White	83.7	80.4	82.0
Black	16.3	17.6	17.0
Other	–	2.0	1.0
Total	100.0	100.0	100.0
Married	70.5	47.8	58.9
Never married	18.2	17.4	17.8
Divorced	9.1	26.1	17.8
Widowed	–	6.5	3.3
Separated	2.3	2.2	2.2
Age			
Mean	32.2	36.2	34.2
SD	11.18	13.40	12.06
Range	18–66	18–70	18–70
Educational Level			
Mean	12.5	12.5	12.5
SD	1.75	1.93	1.83
Range	9–16	9–18	9–18

*Range and age are based on $N = 51$ for women and $N = 49$ for men. Marital status and educational level are based on $N = 46$ for women and $N = 44$ for men.

APPENDIX III
MEANS AND STANDARD DEVIATIONS FOR THE SPECIAL SCALES BASED ON THE INDIANA SAMPLE DATA

Means and Standard Deviations for the Indiana Female Subsample*
$N = 51$

Scale	Mean	SD
L	3.82	2.50
TR	1.75	2.02
CLS	1.63	1.31
ME	49.01	7.52
ME(K)	56.00	6.35
Qu	1.77	3.46
2SD	7.39	4.69
2PR	6.00	1.74
2PM	3.18	1.26
2MD	2.55	2.62
2B	2.55	2.15
3DSA	3.59	1.82
3NA	5.80	2.29
3LM	2.86	2.79
3SC	3.82	3.03
3IA	3.24	1.31
4FD	2.86	2.38
4AC	4.49	1.88
4SI	6.88	2.75
4SOA	6.51	3.04
4SEA	4.49	2.77
5C	5.25	1.75
6PI	2.37	2.11

(Continued)

Scale	Mean	SD
6P	2.43	1.64
6PN	3.98	2.15
8SEA	4.02	3.29
8EA	1.29	1.17
8COG	1.14	1.85
8CON	2.16	2.08
8BSE	2.74	2.85
8DIC	1.88	1.88
9AMO	1.61	1.22
9PMA	5.80	1.90
9IMP	3.02	1.64
9EI	3.53	1.51
AMac	23.31	4.58
OH	14.08	3.50
TSC/I	11.10	5.51
TSC/B	6.76	4.89
TSC/S	12.41	5.00
TSC/D	6.49	5.53
TSC/R	7.59	4.55
TSC/T	11.53	6.17
SOC	11.12	5.80
DEP	7.71	5.99
FEM	19.27	3.50
MOR	8.10	4.98
REL	7.00	2.75
AUT	9.33	3.81
PSY	9.33	4.94
ORG	6.69	5.24
FAM	5.47	3.09
HOS	9.22	4.53
PHO	10.41	3.87
HYP	13.88	3.76
HEA	5.63	3.82
I-SP	2.14	1.46
I-RD	1.73	1.49
I-DS	1.02	1.38
I-OC	3.31	1.68
I-SC	3.78	1.86
I-De	3.86	2.09
I-Do	10.04	2.69
S+	3.20	2.56
D-S	10.78	2.66
Ho	21.00	8.05
Astvn	31.00	4.40
WA	11.35	5.44
E/Cy	5.55	2.78
Cn	26.61	4.46

*Norms for the validity measures Qu, TR, and CLS based on the total normative subgroups of 57 females and 53 males, prior to elimination of cases due to elevated scores on TR and CLS. ME is the mean of T-scores for Scales 1 through 4 and 6 through 9 K-uncorrected. ME(K) is the same index with K-corrected T-scores.

Means and Standard Deviations for the Indiana Male Subsample*
$N = 49$

Scale	Mean	SD
L	4.04	2.27
TR	0.75	1.61
CLS	1.54	1.26
ME	49.02	6.79
ME(K)	58.32	5.94
Qu	1.24	2.96
2SD	6.28	3.72
2PR	5.71	2.00
2PM	2.77	0.98
2MD	1.98	1.88
2B	1.90	1.77
3DSA	3.63	2.02
3NA	5.65	2.40
3LM	2.47	1.99
3SC	2.53	2.36
3IA	2.92	1.24
4FD	2.28	1.63
4AC	5.33	1.74
4SI	7.94	2.36
4SOA	5.96	2.78
4SEA	4.59	2.72
5C	4.65	1.68
6PI	2.16	2.09
6P	2.73	1.55
6N	3.53	2.29
8SOA	3.43	3.07
8EA	1.33	1.11
8COG	1.57	1.84
8CON	2.41	2.12
8BSE	2.22	2.67
8DIC	1.75	1.94
9AMO	1.92	1.17
9PMA	5.84	2.23
9IMP	4.12	1.73
9EI	3.84	1.69
AMac	25.08	4.89
OH	13.29	3.35
TSC/I	8.84	5.48
TSC/B	5.45	4.41
TSC/S	12.24	5.55
TSC/D	5.71	5.03
TSC/R	6.63	3.93
TSC/T	10.51	5.77
SOC	9.88	5.51
DEP	7.24	5.28
FEM	9.86	3.52
MOR	6.28	4.86
REL	6.63	2.47

(Continued)

Scale	Mean	SD
AUT	10.82	4.37
ORG	5.26	3.77
FAM	4.41	2.37
HOS	9.45	4.77
PHO	7.24	4.04
HYP	13.98	4.03
HEA	5.75	3.50
Pe	6.92	2.46
I-SP	2.24	1.57
I-RD	1.90	2.43
I-DS	0.71	1.17
I-OC	3.00	1.68
I-SC	3.20	1.85
I-De	3.94	1.65
I-Do	11.29	2.81
S+	2.73	2.51
D-S	10.14	2.75
Ho	21.22	8.16
WA	11.26	4.97
E/Cy	6.08	2.88
Cn	26.14	5.12

Means and Standard Deviations for the Indiana Total Sample
$N = 100$

Scale	Mean	SD
L	3.93	2.38
TR	1.27	1.91
CLS	1.59	1.29
ME	49.02	7.14
ME(K)	57.14	6.24
Qu	1.52	3.23
2SD	6.85	4.25
2PR	5.86	1.87
2PM	2.98	1.15
2MD	2.27	2.29
2B	2.23	1.99
3DSA	3.61	1.91
3NA	5.73	2.33
3LM	2.67	2.42
3SC	3.19	2.79
3IA	3.08	1.28
4FD	2.58	2.06
4AC	4.90	1.85
4SI	7.40	2.61
4SOA	6.24	2.92
4SEA	4.54	2.73
5C	4.96	1.73

(Continued)

Scale	Mean	SD
6PI	2.27	2.09
6P	2.58	1.60
6N	3.76	2.22
8SOA	3.73	3.18
8EA	1.31	1.13
8COG	1.35	1.85
8CON	2.28	2.09
8BSE	2.49	2.76
8DIC	1.82	1.90
9AMO	1.76	1.20
9PMA	5.82	2.06
9IMP	3.56	1.77
9EI	3.68	1.60
AMac	24.18	4.80
OH	13.69	3.43
TSC/I	9.99	5.59
TSC/B	6.12	4.68
TSC/S	12.33	5.25
TSC/D	6.11	5.28
TSC/R	7.12	4.26
TSC/T	11.03	5.97
SOC	10.51	5.67
DEP	7.48	5.63
FEM	14.66	5.88
MOR	7.21	4.98
REL	6.82	2.61
AUT	10.06	4.14
PSY	9.53	5.46
ORG	5.99	4.61
FAM	4.95	2.80
HOS	9.33	4.63
PHO	8.86	4.24
HYP	13.93	3.87
HEA	5.69	3.65
I-SP	2.19	1.51
I-RD	1.81	2.00
I-DS	0.87	1.28
I-OC	3.16	1 68
I-SC	3.50	1.87
I-De	3.90	1.88
I-Do	10.65	2.81
S+	2.97	2.53
D-S	10.47	2.71
Ho	21.11	8.06
WA	11.31	5.19
E/Cy	5.81	2.83
Cn	26.38	4.78

APPENDIX IV
OBVIOUS-SUBTLE RATINGS
FOR THE SPECIAL SCALES

Obvious–Subtle Ratings of Special Scales According to
Christian, Burkhart, and Gynther (1978)

		Items			
		Total	Subtle*	S%	O-S Rating
2B	Brooding	10	0	0	3.77
2MD	Mental Dullness	15	0	0	3.55
2PM	Physical Malfunctioning	11	2	18	2.88
2PR	Psychomotor Retardation	15	7	47	2.75
2SD	Subjective Depression	30	3	1	3.52
3DSA	Denial of Social Anxiety	6	4	67	2.10
3IA	Inhibition of Aggression	7	5	71	2.39
3LM	Lassitude-Malaise	15	1	7	3.31
3NA	Need for Affection	12	5	42	2.44
3SC	Somatic Complaints	17	2	18	3.26
4SEA	Self-Alienation	15	1	7	3.48
4SI	Social Imperturbability	12	8	67	2.36
4SOA	Social Alienation	18	2	11	3.44
4AC	Authority Conflict	11	5	45	2.74
4FD	Familial Discord	11	3	27	3.02
6N	Naivete	9	6	67	2.31
6PI	Persecutory Ideas	17	0	0	4.16
6P	Poignancy	9	1	11	3.32
8COG	Lack of Ego Mastery, Cognitive	10	0	0	3.74
8CON	Lack of Ego Mastery, Conative	14	1	7	3.67
8DIC	Lack of Ego Mastery, Defect of Inhibition and Control	11	0	0	3.90

(Continued)

		Items			
		Total	Subtle*	S%	O-S Rating
8EA	Emotional Alienation	11	1	9	3.91
8OL	Object Loss	32	1	3	3.67
8SOA	Social Alienation	21	0	0	3.74
8BSE	Bizarre Sensory Experiences	20	0	0	3.65
9AMO	Amorality	6	1	17	2.91
9EI	Ego Inflation	9	2	22	3.09
9IMP	Imperturbability	8	5	63	2.28
9PMA	Psychomotor Acceleration	11	4	36	2.75
AUT	Authority Conflict	20	3	15	2.93
DEP	Depression	33	4	12	3.56
FAM	Family Problems	16	3	19	3.12
FEM	Feminine Interests	30	29	97	1.70
HEA	Poor Health	28	7	25	2.91
HOS	Manifest Hostility	27	3	11	3.29
HYP	Hypomania	25	12	48	2.61
MOR	Poor Morale	23	4	17	3.08
ORG	Organic Symptoms	36	6	17	3.18
PHO	Phobias	27	5	19	3.17
PSY	Psychoticism	45	1	2	3.86
REL	Religious Fundamentalism	12	10	83	1.92
SOC	Social Maladjustment	27	12	44	2.56
TSC/A	Autism	23	4	17	3.22
TSC/B	Body Symptoms	32	2	6	3.27
TSC/D	Depression	28	5	18	3.40
TSC/I	Social Introversion	26	12	46	2.56
TSC/R	Resentment	21	4	20	3.19
TSC/S	Suspicion	25	4	16	2.90
TSC/T	Tension	36	0	0	3.48
I-DS	Dissociative Symptoms	8	1	13	3.90
I-OC	Obsessive-Compulsiveness	9	0	0	3.41
I-RD	Severe Reality Distortion	18	1	6	4.11
I-SC†	Self-Concept (male)	12**	0	0	3.55
	(female)	12**	0	0	3.52
I-SP	Sex Problems (male)	14	0	0	3.59
	(female)	12	0	0	3.91
I-De	Dependency	9	5	56	2.65
I-Do	Dominance	17	13	76	2.38
AMac	Alcoholism	51	25	49	2.63
Cn	Control	50	26	52	2.63
Ho	Hostility	50	9	18	2.98
Astvn	Assertiveness (Female)	57	35	61	2.43
OH	Overcontrolled Hostility	31	19	61	2.39
Pe	Pedophilia	24	9	38	2.83
S+	Extreme Suspiciousness	18	3	17	3.66
WA	Work Attitude	37	6	16	3.25
E/Cy	Cynicism (male)	20	4	20	3.42
	(female)	20	4	20	3.46
5C	Conventionality	9	7	78	2.46
D-S	Depression, Subtle	20	14	70	2.21

*Christian, Burkhart, and Gynther (1978) rating of 2.50 or less.
**Eventually revised to 14 items as in Appendix I.
†Discrepancy is a function of Item 74.

APPENDIX V
THE HUMAN COMPUTER PROGRAM

Computer programs designed to analyze an MMPI record and produce a narrative report have been available for more than two decades. The software is copyrighted and otherwise protected so that program developers are able to charge a fee for each narrative record submitted for analysis. As Fowler (1979) has pointed out, an automated narrative report program is "a report similar in content and style to one written by a skilled MMPI interpreter ... the computer ... programmed to follow the steps typically followed by a clinician in analyzing an MMPI protocol" (p. 347). The program consists of a library of statements from which the computer will automatically select the appropriate ones, according to the MMPI record, and print them sequentially. The library is as effective as the knowledge and skill of the programmer permit.

Computerized MMPI programs have been criticized as inflexible, failing to encompass all available respondent information, and having questionable validity (Butcher, 1978). Automation gives a specious aura of scientific accuracy in presumed contrast to the artistry of the clinician. Yet, the program print-out and the clinician's report are essentially the same product.

This appendix presents in essence the text of the initial stage in the writing of a computerized MMPI narrative program, a library of statements based on the content of this book. Since it is intended to be employed directly by the clinician, no further program development is necessary. Subsequent steps can be provided by the clinician. This requires more human labor than the typical computerized program but it also avoids the inflexibility of such programs. The clinician with sufficient skills could actually transform this appendix into a program that is capable of producing an automated narrative report.

I. VALIDITY

THE STATEMENTS IN THIS SECTION ARE APPROPRIATE WITH RE-SPECTIVE RAW SCORE VALUES OF TR + CLS:

a) BELOW 7

Respondent's verbal comprehension is sufficient to furnish a valid record. He/She appears to have responded honestly to the best of his/her ability. This record is considered to be valid.

b) ABOVE 9

Respondent may have been confused due to stress or drug ingestion when this record was completed, leading to mental confusion. Or he/she may lack sufficient verbal comprehension or intellectual capacity to complete the record validly. It is also possible that he/she has simply been uncooperative for some reason. This record is probably invalid. Direct interpretation of symptom scales should not be attempted. Interpretation of this record should be limited to subtle scales (see pages 46–49).

c) IN THE RANGE OF 7 TO 9

The validity of this record cannot be determined. Interpretation should be approached cautiously. Subtle scales are probably subject to interpretation. Symptom scales may be interpretable.

IF MEAN ELEVATION OF CLINICAL SCALES (ME) IS EQUAL TO OR GREATER THAN T75, OR IF THE MEAN ELEVATION IS EQUAL TO OR GREATER THAN T70 AND AT LEAST FOUR CLINICAL SCALES ARE EQUAL TO OR GREATER THAN T70 AND STATEMENT a) UNDER TR + CLS IS APPLICABLE, WRITE:

Respondent presents herself/himself as severely emotionally disturbed. But this presentation is an exaggeration of his/her actual psychological status. Symptom scales must be interpreted cautiously since they may be invalid in view of the respondent's need to "fake bad." However, statements in this report concerning subtle scales may be considered to be reasonably valid. The most probable explanation of the exaggeration of symptoms is that the respondent is urgently seeking psychotherapeutic intervention and is anxious about the possibility of being rejected for treatment. It is also possible that the respondent is acutely psychotic or is a severe Obsessive-Compulsive Disorder or a Borderline Personality Disorder.

II. MAJOR SYMPTOMS

A. Affective

1. Depression

TRYON, STEIN, & CHU DEPRESSION (TSC/D) and WIGGINS DEPRESSION (DEP): When scores are T60 and above, the report usually requires some statement concerning depression as a symptom or condition. The exact statement will depend on the level of TSC/D and DEP and also HARRIS AND LINGOES 2PR, 2MD, 2PM compared to 2SD and on MOR and I-SC.

Statements that clinical depression is present require that MOR and I-SC be significantly elevated, ordinarily at least in the same range as TSC/D and DEP.

IF THESE NEGATIVE SELF-CONCEPT SCALES ARE NOT SIGNIFICANTLY ELEVATED, THE PRESENCE OF CLINICAL DEPRESSION IS CONTRAINDICATED, EVEN IF TSC/D AND/OR DEP ARE ELEVATED, WRITE:

Respondent is chronically unhappy because of circumstances in his/her environment and/or in interpersonal relationships that he/she feels powerless to control. Or, he/she may have a progressive, deteriorating or fatal disease.

IF MOR AND I-SC ARE SIGNIFICANTLY ELEVATED AND BOTH TSC/D AND DEP ARE IN THE RANGE T65–69, OR ONE IS IN THAT RANGE AND THE OTHER IN THE RANGE T60–64, WRITE:

Respondent is moderately depressed.

IF BOTH TSC/D AND DEP ARE IN THE RANGE OF T65–69, WRITE:

Respondent is moderately depressed.

IF EITHER TSC/D OR DEP IS IN THE RANGE T60 TO 64, AND 2 OR MORE OF THESE CRITICAL ITEMS ARE ENDORSED:

Much of the time I feel as if I have done something wrong or evil. (106)
I believe my sins are unpardonable. (209)
Most of the time I wish I were dead. (339)
I deserve severe punishment for my sins. (413)

WRITE:

Respondent is moderately depressed.

IF BOTH TSC/D AND DEP ARE T70 OR ABOVE, OR IF ONE IS T70 OR ABOVE AND THE OTHER IS IN THE RANGE T65–69, WRITE:

Respondent is seriously clinically depressed.

2. Suicidal Tendency

IF YOU HAVE WRITTEN THAT THE RESPONDENT IS SERIOUSLY CLINICALLY DEPRESSED AND HARRIS & LINGOES 2PR IS BELOW T60, AND ESPECIALLY IF THE FOLLOWING ITEMS ARE ENDORSED:

Most of the time I wish I were dead. (339)
The future seems hopeless to me. (526)

IMMEDIATELY FOLLOWING THE STATEMENT OF SEVERE DEPRES-SION, WRITE:

Respondent may be suicidal. Suicidal threats or gestures should be taken seriously and the possibility of suicide should be carefully investigated.

3. Dysthymia-Anhedonia

IF DEP, TSC/D AND 2SD ARE BELOW T60 AND THE WIENER & HAR-MON DEPRESSION-SUBTLE SCALE (D-S) IS ABOVE T60, WRITE:

Respondent is not depressed in the clinical sense but is chronically unhappy with his/her life space. He/She seldom regards himself/herself as in a good mood, rarely is elated, and is often cross and irritable. Such respondents are not helped by anti-depressive medication.

4. Hypomania

For interpretation in the section, refer to Personality Traits and Behavior Patterns Features section in the Extroversion subsection (III. B)

B. Anxiety

1. Trait Anxiety

IF THE TRYON, STEIN, & CHU TENSION SCALE (TSC/T) IS IN THE RANGE T60–69, WRITE:

The respondent has a moderately high trait anxiety level and may be considered to be a "worrier" but behavior is not seriously negatively affected.

IF TSC/T IS T70 OR ABOVE, WRITE:

The respondent has a high trait anxiety level which probably interferes with his/her functioning.

MENTION RELEVANT ITEM ENDORSEMENTS:

I work under a great deal of tension. (13)
I frequently find myself worrying about something. (217)
I have periods of such great restlessness that I cannot sit long in a chair. (238)
I believe I am no more nervous than most others. (F) (242)
I feel anxiety about something or someone almost all the time. (337)
I have certainly had more than my share of things to worry about. (338)
I am usually calm and not easily upset. (F) (407)
I worry quite a bit over possible misfortunes. (431)
I must admit that I have at times been worried beyond reason over something that really did not matter. (499)
Several times a week I feel as if something dreadful is about to happen. (543)

2. Phobia

IF A STATEMENT HAS BEEN WRITTEN UNDER TRAIT ANXIETY AND THE WIGGINS PHOBIAS SCALE (PHO) IS T62 OR ABOVE FOR MALES AND T65 OR ABOVE FOR FEMALES, WRITE:

Not surprisingly, the respondent has a fair amount of phobic anxiety.

IF A STATEMENT HAS not BEEN WRITTEN UNDER TRAIT ANXIETY AND PHO IS T62 OR ABOVE FOR MEN AND T65 OR ABOVE FOR WOMEN, WRITE:

The respondent has a fair amount of phobic anxiety despite having a normal trait anxiety level. This area should be investigated further.

IF A STATEMENT HAS BEEN WRITTEN UNDER PHOBIA, MENTION SPECIFIC ITEM ENDORSEMENTS:

The sight of blood neither frightens me nor makes me sick. (F) (128)
I do not worry about catching diseases. (F) (131)
I am afraid when I look down from a high place. (166)
I am not afraid to handle money. (F) (169)
I do not have a great fear of snakes. (F) (176)
I get anxious and upset when I have to make a short trip away from home. (351)
I am not afraid of fire. (F) (367/400)
Lightning is one of my fears. (385/469)
I am afraid to be alone in the dark. (388/481)
A windstorm terrifies me. (392/502)
I have no fear of water. (F) (401)
I am often afraid of the dark. (480)
I dread the thought of an earthquake. (492)
I am afraid of finding myself in a closet or small closed place. (494)
Dirt frightens or disgusts me. (510)
I have no fear of spiders. (F) (522)
I am not afraid of mice. (F) (539)
I am afraid of being alone in a wide-open place. (553)

(Note: Some PHOBIAS SCALE items do NOT refer to specific phobias.)

3. Dissociation

IF THE INDIANA DISSOCIATIVE SYMPTOMS SCALE (I-DS) IS T70 OR ABOVE, WRITE:

Respondent admits to behaviors and experiences that may be pathognomonic of a dissociative state or an hysterical illness, or they may suggest organic involvement.

MENTION RELEVANT ITEM ENDORSEMENTS:

At times I have fits of laughing and crying that I cannot control. (22)
My soul sometimes leaves my body. (50)
I have had periods in which I carried on activities without knowing later what I had been doing. (156)
I have had attacks in which I could not control my movements or speech but in which I knew what was going on around me. (194)
I have had blank spells in which my activities were interrupted and I did not know what was going on around me. (251)
I often feel as if things were not real. (345)
I have had some very unusual religious experiences. (420)
I have never seen a vision. (F) (464)

IF HARRIS & LINGOES 8 BIZARRE SENSORY EXPERIENCES SCALE (8BSE) IS ABOVE T70, WRITE:

The possibility that one of these conditions exists is supported by the respondent's claim that he/she has had some peculiar sensory or sensorimotor experiences.

C. Psychosis

1. Severe Reality Distortion

The presence of a psychosis in the respondent cannot be reliably determined by a verbal inventory like the MMPI. Yet, there are various possible clues that are at least suggestive and worth mentioning in a report. Always carefully qualify. Labeling a respondent as psychotic should not be done casually. The scales that are most useful in providing clues for psychoticism are:

8BSE, PSY, S+ and especially I-RD.

The problem is how to write the rules that would cover the interfacing among these scales for all respondents. A further complication is that there is a cluster of items in the PSY scale that overlap with the various alienation scales. The level of those scales must be considered in interpreting the PSY scale. Still another problem is that a plurality of definitely psychotic statements on the MMPI are paranoid indicators. Many psychoses have a paranoid component but some do not and may not be singled out by any of the four scales used to diagnose psychoticism.

If INDIANA SEVERE REALITY DISTORTION SCALE (I-RD) IS IN THE RANGE OF T60–69—WRITE:

Respondent admits to symptoms that are usually considered to reflect the existence of a psychosis, such as hallucinations.

Then make specific reference to the I-RD items that have been endorsed:

Evil spirits possess me at times. (27)
I have had very peculiar and strange experiences. (33)
When I am with people I am bothered by hearing very queer things. (48)
My soul sometimes leaves my body. (50)
I see things or animals or people around me that others do not see. (66)
I believe I am being plotted against. (121)
I believe I am being followed. (123)
Someone has been trying to poison me. (151)
I commonly hear voices without knowing where they come from. (184)

There are persons who are trying to steal my thoughts and ideas. (200)
Someone has control over my mind. (275)
At one or more times in my life I felt that someone was making me do things by hypnotizing me. (291)
Peculiar odors come to me at times. (334)
I often feel as if things were not real. (345)
I have strange and peculiar thoughts. (349)
I hear strange things when I am alone. (350)
I have never seen a vision. (F) (464)
I am a special agent of God. (476)

IF I-RD IS IN THE RANGE T60–69 AND 8BSE IS IN THE RANGE OF T60–69—ADD:

Furthermore, the respondent states that he/she has some unusual and peculiar sensory and sensorimotor experiences that might also be indicative of a psychotic process.

IF I-RD IS ABOVE T69—WRITE:

Respondent admits to a large number of symptoms that are usually considered to reflect the existence of a psychosis, such as hallucinations and peculiar or bizarre experiences.

IF I-RD IS BELOW T59, LOOK AT WIGGINS PSYCHOTICISM SCALE (PSY).

IF PSY IS T65 OR ABOVE BUT IS LESS THAN 10 T-SCORE POINTS ABOVE HARRIS & LINGOES 4 SOCIAL ALIENATION AND 8 SOCIAL ALIENATION (4SOA AND 8SOA), THEN NO STATEMENT FOR PSY IS WARRANTED. IF PSY IS T65 OR ABOVE AND IS MORE THAN 10 T-SCORE POINTS ABOVE 4SOA AND 8SOA—WRITE:

Respondent admits to a number of symptoms that are usually considered to reflect the existence of a psychosis such as unexplained loss of control and having strange or peculiar experiences.

Following any of the above statements based on I-RD and/or PSY ADD:

Despite the indicators of a possible psychosis, a definite diagnosis cannot be made. Additional diagnostic investigation is suggested.

IF I-RD OR PSY IS T70 OR ABOVE—ADD:

Diagnosis of a psychotic process by means of a verbal inventory must always be tentative. Nevertheless, if the respondent's verbal comprehension is adequate and the respondent responded truthfully, there is a reasonable probability that the respondent is psychotic.

2. Paranoia

IF S+ IS IN THE RANGE T60–69, WRITE:

Respondent gives indications of paranoid ideation.

IF S+ IS T70 OR ABOVE, WRITE:

Respondent is clearly paranoid and delusional. *Specifically note endorsement of any of the following items:*

Evil spirits possess me at times. (27)
I believe I am being plotted against. (121)
I believe I am being followed. (123)
Someone has been trying to poison me. (151)
There are persons who are trying to steal my thoughts and ideas. (200)
Someone has control over my mind. (275)
At one or more times in my life I felt that someone was making me do things by hypnotizing me. (291)
Someone has been trying to influence my mind. (293)
People say insulting and vulgar things about me. (364)
I am bothered by people outside, on streetcars, in stores, etc., watching me. (448)

3. Cognitive Disturbance

IF HARRIS & LINGOES 2 MENTAL DULLNESS (2MD) IS IN THE RANGE T60–69 WRITE:

Respondent complains of difficulty with concentration, memory and logical thinking.

IF 2MD IS ABOVE T69, WRITE:

Respondent complains of severe difficulty with concentration, memory and logical thinking and has probably lost all confidence in his/her ability to function in the cognitive sphere.

IF A STATEMENT HAS BEEN WRITTEN FOR 2MD, EXAMINE HARRIS & LINGOES 8 LACK OF EGO MASTERY, COGNITIVE (8COG). IF IT IS IN THE RANGE T60–69, WRITE:

Respondent is also troubled by being unable to avoid thoughts that he/she considers irrational.

IF 8COG IS ABOVE T69, ADD:

He/She may believe that the cognitive dysfunction is an indication that he/she is, or is becoming, psychotic.

IF A STATEMENT HAS BEEN WRITTEN FOR 2MD, RE-EXAMINE TR AND CLS. IF TR + CLS IS EQUAL TO, OR GREATER THAN 7, AMEND THE VALIDITY STATEMENT AS FOLLOWS:

Responses in the record indicate that the respondent was probably confused at the time that the inventory was administered.

D. Anger

1. Manifest Hostility

IF WIGGINS MANIFEST HOSTILITY SCALE (HOS) IS IN THE RANGE T58–64, WRITE:

Respondent has angry feelings and hostile impulses. He/She may tend to be irritable, impatient, argumentative, competitive and overly assertive.

IF HOS IS T65 OR ABOVE, ADD TO THE STATEMENT ABOVE:

He/She may be experiencing difficulty in controlling these hostile feelings.

IF A STATEMENT ABOVE HAS BEEN WRITTEN AND THE TRYON, STEIN, & CHU RESENTMENT SCALE (TSC/R) IS IN THE RANGE T65–69, ADD:

He/She is especially likely to resent being asked to assume responsibilities and is apt to respond by being cross, verbally abusive and/or passive-aggressive.

IF A STATEMENT UNDER HOS ABOVE HAS BEEN WRITTEN AND TSC/R IS T70 OR ABOVE, SUBSTITUTE FOR THE ABOVE STATEMENT:

Most of his/her hostility stems from being asked to assume responsibilities. His/Her resentment is apt to be expressed by being cross and verbally abusive. However, he/she may react with physical violence or destructive behavior.

IF A STATEMENT UNDER HOS HAS NOT BEEN WRITTEN AND TSC/R IS IN THE RANGE T62–69, WRITE:

Respondent has some angry feelings and hostile impulses that are typically adolescent. He/She resents demands being made of him/her and is apt to respond by being cross, verbally abusive and passive-aggressive.

IF A STATEMENT UNDER HOS HAS NOT BEEN WRITTEN AND TSC/R IS T70 OR ABOVE, ELIMINATE THE TERM "PASSIVE-AGGRESSIVE" AND SUBSTITUTE:

... may react by being physically violent and/or destructive.

IF HOS AND TSC/R ARE BOTH T40 OR BELOW, FOR MALES IN THE AGE RANGE 15–45 YEARS, WRITE:

Respondent tends to be submissive, unassertive, somewhat anergic and is probably suggestible and easily manipulated.

2. Overcontrolled Hostility and Intermittent Explosive Disorder

IF THE OVERCONTROLLED HOSTILITY SCALE (OH) IS T65 OR ABOVE, WRITE:

Respondent tends to strongly repress hostile feelings so that he/she may appear placid even when provoked. He/She may be regarded by intimate acquaintances as quiet, reserved and unassuming. On rare occasions, he/she may give vent to a brief outburst of violent behavior. Respondent may be a case of Intermittent Explosive Disorder.

IF OH IS T65 OR ABOVE AND A STATEMENT HAS BEEN WRITTEN UNDER THE ANGER SECTION, INSTEAD OF THE STATEMENT ABOVE, WRITE:

Respondent regards any expression of anger as improper and inappropriate which causes conflict with his/her need to express those feelings. He/She may therefore experience some guilt about the expression of anger and will have a strong tendency to externalize blame for it.

E. Health Concerns

HEALTH CONCERNS SCALES SHOULD BE EXAMINED IN THE FOL-LOWING ORDER:

1. Tryon, Stein & Chu Body Symptoms Scale (TSC/B)
2. Wiggins Poor Health Scale (HEA)
3. Wiggins Organic Symptoms Scale (ORG)

IF TSC/B IS IN THE RANGE T60–69, WRITE:

Respondent is anxious about his/her physical health. He/She expresses a variety of concerns, primarily minor complaints commonly associated with emotional illnesses, such as vague pains, sleep disorder, easy fatigability, anergia and minor gastrointestinal disorders.

IF TSC/B IS T70 OR ABOVE, WRITE:

Respondent is preoccupied with his/her physical health to an extent that might be considered hypochondriacal. He/She expresses a wide variety of concerns, primarily minor complaints commonly associated with emotional illnesses, such as vague pains, sleep disorder, easy fatigability, anergia and minor gastrointestinal disorders.

IF NO STATEMENT FOR TSC/B IS WARRANTED, EXAMINE HEA. IF HEA IS IN THE RANGE T60–69, WRITE:

Respondent expresses a variety of physical health concerns, primarily complaints of gastrointestinal disorders.

IF HEA IS T70 OR ABOVE, ADD THE WORD "wide" BEFORE "variety" IN THE PRECEDING STATEMENT.
IF ORG IS IN THE RANGE T60–65, WRITE:

Respondent (also) complains of some sensory and motor disorders that may have a central nervous system etiology or may be pathognomonic of a dissociative or hysterical disorder. Further investigation is suggested.

IF ORG IS T66 OR ABOVE, SUBSTITUTE THE WORD "many" FOR "some" IN THE ABOVE STATEMENT.

III. PERSONALITY TRAITS
AND BEHAVIOR PATTERNS

A. Social Adjustment

This dimension is measured by five scales:

Harris & Lingoes
    Denial of Social Anxiety (3DSA)
    Social Imperturbability (4SI)
    Imperturbability (9IMP)
Wiggins Social Maladjustment Scale (SOC)
Tryon, Stein & Chu Social Introversion Scale (TSC/I)

IF THE SUM OF THE T-SCORES FOR 3DSA, 4SI AND 9IMP FALLS IN THE RANGE 130–160, WRITE:

Respondent claims that he/she is reasonably comfortable in social situations, in meeting new people and interacting interpersonally.

IF THE SUM OF T-SCORES FOR 3DSA, 4SI AND 9IMP IS ABOVE 160, WRITE:

Respondent claims to be very comfortable in social situations, seeks them for pleasure and enjoys making new friends.

IF THE SUM OF THE T-SCORES FOR 3DSA, 4SI AND 9IMP FALLS IN THE RANGE 120–129, WRITE:

Respondent is somewhat socially anxious. He/She tends to be uncomfortable with interpersonal relations and with meeting new people and tries to avoid such circumstances.

IF THE SUM OF THE T-SCORES FOR 3DSA, 4SI AND 9IMP FALLS BELOW 120, WRITE:

Respondent is acutely socially anxious. He/She is highly uncomfortable with interpersonal relations, strongly dislikes meeting new people and will go to considerable lengths to avoid such circumstances.

Note: SOC and TSC/I ordinarily co-fluctuate negatively with the social anxiety triad. When the latter is pathologically low and the former pathologically high, the term *avoidant* may be appropriately applied to the respondent. SOC and TSC/I normally co-fluctuate as well, due to a heavy overlap of items in addition to similar intent. Interpretively, it is reasonable to consider them as yoked. If the scores are sufficiently disparate to create an interpretive problem, rely on SOC since it has many more items.

IF SOC AND TSC/I ARE IN THE RANGE T60–69, WRITE:

Respondent tends to be shy, self-conscious, reticent and easily embarrassed. He/She tends to withdraw under stress, especially if it involves interpersonal relations.

IF SOC-TSC/I ARE T70 OR ABOVE, WRITE:

Respondent is extremely shy, very self-conscious, reticent and easily embarrassed. He/She has a strong tendency to withdraw under stress, especially if it involves interpersonal relations. He/She may be considered to have avoidant tendencies.

B. Extroversion

IF WIGGINS HYPOMANIA SCALE (HYP) IS IN THE RANGE T60–69, WRITE:

Respondent is an outgoing person, who usually appears cheerful and enthusiastic. He/She may be restless, emotionally labile and easily excited. These characteristics do not necessarily reflect psychopathology.

IF HYP IS T70 OR ABOVE, WRITE:

Respondent is an outgoing person who usually appears cheerful and enthusiastic. He/She is likely to be easily excitable, restless, impulsive and emotionally labile. This pattern may reflect an immaturity that could interfere with the respondent's pursuing an orderly existence.

IF HARRIS & LINGOES 9 PSYCHOMOTOR ACCELERATION (9PMA) IS IN THE RANGE T60–69 (unless respondent is a male under age 30), WRITE:

Respondent's optimum stimulation level is above average. He/She will seek more than the usual amount of excitement and social stimulation.

(Note: for males under age 30, this statement requires at least T75).

IF 9PMA IS T70 OR ABOVE (unless respondent is a male under age 30), WRITE:

Respondent has an unusually high optimum stimulation level. He/She is likely to be unhappy without excitement and social stimulation on a regular basis.

(Note: for males under age 30, this statement requires at least T80).

C. Social Hypersensitivity

IF HARRIS & LINGOES 6 POIGNANCY (6P) IS T65 OR ABOVE, WRITE:

Respondent views himself/herself as unusually sensitive and highstrung, and believes that he/she has more intense feelings than other people.

D. Alienation

IF 4SOA AND 8SOA ARE IN THE RANGE T60–69, OR IF AT LEAST ONE IS T65 OR ABOVE, WRITE:

Respondent feels misunderstood, isolated, different from others, and without a viable social support system.

IF EITHER 4SOA OR 8SOA IS T70 OR ABOVE AND THE OTHER IS AT LEAST T60, WRITE:

Respondent has a sense of being totally estranged from society. He/She feels misunderstood, isolated, different from others and discriminated against. He/She lacks a viable social support system.

E. Authority Conflict

Authority conflict is measured by Harris & Lingoes 4 Authority Conflict Scale (4AC) and Wiggins Authority Conflict Scale (AUT). These are usually positively correlated. However, in some respondents, AUT may be elevated alone. This disparity can be interpreted.

IF BOTH 4AC AND AUT ARE IN THE RANGE T60–65, WRITE:

Respondent tends to be a somewhat rebellious person but not to an extent that this tendency would hinder him/her in his/her occupational or social life.

IF AUT IS T65 OR ABOVE AND 4AC IS BELOW 60, ADD TO THE ABOVE STATEMENT:

Respondent is probably unaware of his/her rebellious tendency.

IF 4AC AND/OR AUT IS T70 OR ABOVE, WRITE:

Respondent tends to be a rebellious person who may experience difficulties in home, school or community because of his/her negativistic attitude toward rules and authority figures.

IF RESPONDENT IS A MALE UNDER AGE 21, ADD:

However, his rebelliousness may be a developmental phase that will become modified in later life.

F. Suspiciousness and Social Distrust

Scales involved in this dimension, usually an aspect of antisocial personality, are the Tryon, Stein & Chu Suspicion Scale (TSC/S), Eichman Cynicism scale (E/Cy), and the Cook & Medley Hostility Scale (Ho).

IF TSC/S IS T65 OR ABOVE, WRITE:

Respondent is a suspicious person who questions the motives and intentions of others and tends to be doubtful about the motives of authority figures and the reasons for rules.

IF E/Cy IS T65 OR ABOVE, WRITE:

Respondent believes that the behavior of others is motivated entirely by self-interest and therefore no one can be trusted, especially if they claim to have altruistic intentions.

IF Ho IS IN THE RANGE T60–69, WRITE:

Respondent is an angry, critical, distrustful person who suspects the motivation of others and is likely to be calculating and vigilant in his/her dealings with them.

IF Ho IS T70 OR ABOVE, ADD TO THE PREVIOUS STATEMENT:

He/She is especially critical of intimates and other supporting persons, tends to find them inadequate and may have consequent depressive episodes. These respondents are inclined to engage in behaviors like smoking and excessive use of alcohol and tend to have unhealthy eating habits.

G. Compulsivity

The MMPI lacks the necessary items to permit a diagnosis of Obsessive-Compulsive Disorder. The Indiana Obsessive-Compulsiveness Scale (I-OC) can be used only to make some limited statements.

IF I-OC IS IN THE RANGE T60–T74, WRITE:

Respondent has an obsessive-compulsive tendency and probably some minor compulsions but these tendencies do not appear to interfere with his/her daily functioning.

IF STATEMENTS HAVE BEEN WRITTEN UNDER PSYCHOSIS (II, C) AND I-OC IS ABOVE T75, ADD TO THE STATEMENTS UNDER PSYCHOSIS (II, C):

Patient's symptoms include a ritualistic tendency which may appear as bizarre behavior.

H. Dependency and Dominance

I-De and I-Do respectively measure these two characteristics. They have a strong negative relationship especially when one or the other is clearly elevated.

IF I-De IS T60 OR ABOVE OR IF I-De IS AT ANY LEVEL BUT IS AT LEAST 15 T-SCORE POINTS ABOVE I-Do, WRITE:

Respondent has strong dependency needs and is characterized by a lack of self-confidence and an inability to make decisions. His/Her self-esteem depends largely on external sources and he/she will usually subordinate his/her desires to those of persons on whom he/she depends.

IF I-Do IS IN THE RANGE T60–69 OR IF I-Do IS AT ANY LEVEL BUT IS AT LEAST 15 T-SCORE POINTS ABOVE I-De, WRITE:

Respondent claims to be confident, self-assured and assertive. He/She often has strong opinions and needs to dominate his/her usual milieus.

IF I-Do IS T70 OR ABOVE, WRITE:

Respondent claims to be confident and able to control various situations but these claims probably represent denial of feelings of inadequacy and dependency needs.

(NOTE: IF RESPONDENT IS FEMALE, SEE ALSO SECTION III, L).

I. Family Conflict

This dimension is measured by Harris & Lingoes 4 Family Discord Scale (4FD) and Wiggins Family Problems Scale (FAM). They are highly positively correlated.

IF 4FD IS T65 OR ABOVE, WRITE:

Respondent regards his/her home life and family situation as unpleasant and lacking in warmth and affection.

IF FAM IS T60 OR ABOVE, WRITE:

Respondent is dissatisfied with his/her home situation and may find it stressful due to the behavior of some family members.

NOTE: IF THE RESPONDENT LIVES WITH HIS/HER PARENTS, AND A STATEMENT HAS BEEN WRITTEN UNDER FAMILY CONFLICT, ADD:

Respondent has probably considered leaving home a number of times.

J. Alcoholism/Drug Abuse

IF A MALE RESPONDENT ATTAINS A RAW SCORE OF 27, OR A FEMALE ATTAINS A RAW SCORE OF 25 ON THE MacANDREWS ALCOHOLISM SCALE (AMac), WRITE:

Respondent is involved, or is at strong risk of becoming involved, in excessive use of alcohol or other substances.

NOTE: IF THE PRECEDING COMMENT WAS WRITTEN *AND* IF RE-SPONDENT HAS *NOT* ENDORSED EITHER ITEM, "Except by doctor's orders I never take drugs or sleeping powders" (466) OR THE ITEM "I have used alcohol excessively," (215) WRITE:

Respondent may be denying or concealing this problem or it may not yet have manifested itself.

K. Sexual Problems

IF THE INDIANA SEX PROBLEMS SCALE (I-SP) IS IN THE RANGE T60–69, WRITE:

Respondent may have a problem in the sexual area.

IF I-SP IS T70 OR ABOVE, WRITE:

Respondent has a problem in the sexual area.

FOR CLUES TO THE SPECIFIC PROBLEM, EXAMINE I-SP CONTENT, ESPECIALLY THE FOLLOWING ITEMS:

I am strongly attracted by members of my own sex. (69)
I have often wished I were a girl (Or if you are a girl) I have never been sorry that I am a girl. (male T; female F) (74)
I have never indulged in any unusual sex practices. (F) (133)
I am attracted by members of the opposite sex. (F) (430)
Sexual things disgust me. (470)
There is something wrong with my sex organs. (519)

IF THE PEDOPHILIA SCALE (Pe) IS T65 OR ABOVE, WRITE:

Respondent probably has a paraphilia such as exhibitionism, voyeurism, or pedophilia.

IF Pe IS T65 OR ABOVE AND RESPONDENT HAS ENDORSED THE ITEM, "I am very strongly attracted by members of my own sex," (69) ESPECIALLY IF HE/SHE HAS *NOT* ENDORSED THE ITEM, "I am attracted by members of the opposite sex," (430) SUBSTITUTE FOR THE STATEMENT ABOVE:

Respondent appears to be a dystonic homosexual.

L. Gender Identity

For Female Respondents

IF WIGGINS FEMININE INTERESTS SCALE (FEM) IS IN THE RANGE T40–59 AND RESPONDENT HAS LESS THAN 14 YEARS OF FORMAL EDUCATION, WRITE:

Respondent has normal interests in occupations and activities that are stereotypically feminine and a corresponding lack of interest in masculine pursuits.

IF FEM IS IN THE RANGE T35–59 AND RESPONDENT HAS MORE THAN 14 YEARS OF FORMAL EDUCATION, WRITE:

Respondent's interest in feminine occupations and activities is normal for her educational level.

IF FEM IS IN THE RANGE T60–69, WRITE:

Respondent has more than average interest in occupations and activities that are stereotypically feminine and a corresponding lack of interest in masculine pursuits.

IF FEM IS T70 OR ABOVE, WRITE:

Respondent claims to have an unusually great interest in stereotypical feminine occupations and activities. Such a claim is sufficiently remarkable that the possibility of denial must be considered. Respondent may have doubts about her feminine identity.

IF FEM IS BELOW T40 OR T35 FOR RESPONDENTS WITH 14 YEARS OF FORMAL EDUCATION OR MORE, WRITE:

Respondent expresses less than normal interest in activities that are stereotypically feminine. The possibility of a gender identity problem should be considered.

IF A STATEMENT HAS BEEN WRITTEN IN THIS SECTION INDICATING THAT RESPONDENT'S INTERESTS ARE NORMAL AND ASTVN IS T65 OR ABOVE, WRITE:

Respondent is a person who tends to express her views and feelings openly. Such a tendency is not necessarily associated with a dominance need, hostility or a gender identity problem (CHECK WITH STATEMENTS UNDER SECTION II, D, 1 AND SECTION III, E, H AND K FOR POSSIBLE MODIFICATION OF THIS STATEMENT).

IF FEM IS BELOW T40 OR BELOW T35 FOR A RESPONDENT WITH 14 YEARS OF FORMAL EDUCATION OR MORE AND ASTVN IS T65 OR ABOVE, WRITE:

Respondent is a person who tends to express her views and feelings openly. She may have a gender identity problem (CHECK WITH STATEMENTS UNDER SECTION II, D, 1 AND SECTION II, E, H AND K AND INDIVIDUAL ITEM ENDORSEMENTS IN I-SP FOR POSSIBLE CONFIRMATION OF THIS STATEMENT).

For Male Respondents

IF FEM IS T59 OR LESS AND RESPONDENT HAS LESS THAN 14 YEARS OF FORMAL EDUCATION, WRITE:

Respondent expresses normal interest in occupations and activities that are stereotypically masculine and a corresponding lack of interest in feminine pursuits.

IF FEM IS IN THE RANGE T51–65 AND RESPONDENT HAS 14 YEARS OF FORMAL EDUCATION OR MORE, WRITE:

Respondent's interest in masculine occupations and in feminine activities is normal for his educational level.

IF FEM IS ABOVE T59 FOR A RESPONDENT WITH LESS THAN 14 YEARS OF FORMAL EDUCATION, OR ABOVE T65 FOR A RESPONDENT WITH AT LEAST 14 YEARS OF FORMAL EDUCATION, WRITE:

Respondent has a below average interest in occupations and activities that are stereotypically masculine and a high interest in feminine pursuits. The possibility of inversion should be investigated.

NOTE: IF A STATEMENT HAS BEEN WRITTEN FOR I-SP AND/OR Pe, CALL ATTENTION TO IT AT THIS POINT.

M. Religious Fundamentalism

IF WIGGINS RELIGIOUS FUNDAMENTALISM SCALE (REL) IS T58 OR ABOVE, WRITE:

Respondent claims to be a devoutly religious person who probably has fundamentalist religious beliefs and is likely to be intolerant of the religious convictions of others.

N. Morality and Virtue

This pattern is reflected in three Harris & Lingoes Scales. The Lie Scale (L) and the Conventionality Scale (5C) may also be elevated.

Need for Affection (3NA) (high score)
Naivete (6N) (high score)
Amorality (9AMO) (low score)

As a rule, 3NA and 6N will be positively correlated and 9AMO will be negatively correlated with them. When it is not, refer to the section on Inconsistent or Conflictual Responding.

IF THE T-SCORES FOR 3NA AND 6N SUM TO AT LEAST 125 AND NEITHER REACHES T70 (9AMO IS EXPECTED TO BE T45 OR BELOW), WRITE:

Respondent presents himself/herself as optimistic, trusting and uncritical. He/She views the environment as benign and believes that others are honest and reasonable. These perceptions are likely to be a consequence of the respondent's greater than average need for affection and friendship.

IF EITHER OR BOTH 3NA AND 6N ARE T70 OR ABOVE, ADD THE FOLLOWING TO THE ABOVE STATEMENT:

However, it is possible that these claims reflect denial of hostile or negative feelings.

DO NOT WRITE ANY OF THE ABOVE STATEMENTS UNDER Morality and Virtue IF THE RESPONDENT IS LESS THAN 60 YEARS OF AGE AND HAS EIGHT YEARS OF FORMAL SCHOOLING OR LESS AND THE LIE SCALE (L) IS T62 OR ABOVE. INSTEAD, WRITE:

Respondent claims to be a moral, virtuous, trusting person. However, these claims appear to be a consequence of defensiveness in responding and may also reflect denial of hostile or negative feelings.

IV. THE PERSONALITY DISORDERS

The interpretive process in this section differs somewhat from the approach in earlier sections. The reason for the differences is inherent in the nature of personality disorders; they typically contain several of the traits or symptoms in Section III and sometimes also traits and symptoms in Section II. The interpretive statements must be written to be comprehensive enough to cover the multiple special scale markers for each personality disorder. Another difference is the application of the personality disorder supplementary item sets (Table 5.4), in accordance with the scales-plus-items approach.

Scales or clusters may be included in the interpretive guidelines whose presence though common, is not found invariably. In such instances, the interpretive guideline may make use of the incidence terms *usually, frequently, often, sometimes*, which are ordered according to incidence from most to least.

It will be rare for *all* of the interpretive guidelines to be met for any personality disorder. As always in clinical practice, a final decision is contingent upon other sources of information as well as formal test data.

When many, but not all of the interpretive criteria are met for any personality disorder, the clinician should consider the possibility of a mixed, atypical or not specified personality disorder and examine criteria for other personality disorders.

A. Antisocial Personality Disorder

(1) IF THE ANTISOCIAL SUPPLEMENTARY ITEM SET (Table 5.4) IS AT LEVEL III OR ABOVE, INCLUDING ENDORSEMENT OF CONDUCT DISORDERED LIFE HISTORY ITEMS AND (2) AMORALITY IS PRESENT (9AMO IS IN THE RANGE OF T67 OR ABOVE, AND T-SCORES FOR 3NA AND 6N SUM TO 90 OR LESS AND NEITHER EXCEEDS T54), OFTEN ACCOMPANIED BY UNCONVENTIONAL ATTITUDES AND VALUES (5C IS T40 OR BELOW) AND OFTEN BY AUTHORITY CONFLICT (4AC AND/OR AUT IS T70 OR ABOVE) AND (3) IRRITABILITY AND AGGRESSIVENESS USUALLY ARE EVIDENT (HOS IS T65 OR ABOVE AND/OR TSC/R IS T70 OR ABOVE, AND I-Do EXCEEDS I-De BY A T-SCORE DIFFERENCE OF 20 POINTS OR MORE) AND (4) SOCIAL DISTRUST AND SUSPICIOUSNESS ARE USUALLY PROMINENT ALONG WITH SOCIAL ALIENATION AND FAMILY CONFLICT (T-SCORES FOR TSC/S, E/Cy AND Ho AVERAGE 65 OR ABOVE; 4SOA AND 8SOA ARE T60–69; FAM IS T60 OR ABOVE AND 4FD IS T65 OR MORE) AND (5) THE INDIVIDUAL

FREQUENTLY ACTS ON IMPULSE (HYP IS T60 OR ABOVE, AND 9PMA IS T65 OR ABOVE), WHICH IS EXACERBATED BY DRUG ABUSE, WRITE:

Respondent possesses the cardinal characteristics of the antisocial personality disorder.

B. Paranoid Personality Disorder

(1) IF THE PARANOID SUPPLEMENTARY ITEM SET (Table 5.4) IS AT LEVEL III OR ABOVE AND (2) EXTREME SUSPICION AND SENSITIVITY ARE PRESENT (USUALLY S+ IS IN THE RANGE T60–69 AND 6P IS T65 OR ABOVE) AND (3) SOCIAL DISTRUST, ALIENATION, AMORALITY, UNCONVENTIONAL ATTITUDES, AND AUTHORITY AND FAMILY CONFLICT ALL ARE FREQUENTLY PRESENT (TSC/S, E/Cy AND Ho AVERAGE T65 OR ABOVE; AND 4SOA OR 8SOA IS T70 OR ABOVE AND THE OTHER IS AT LEAST T60; 9AMO IS IN THE RANGE OF T60–69, AND 3NA AND 6N SUM TO 90 OR LESS AND NEITHER EXCEEDS T50; 5C IS T40 OR BELOW; 4AC AND/OR AUT IS T70 OR ABOVE; AND 4FD IS T65 OR ABOVE, AND FAM IS T60 OR ABOVE) AND (4) TENDENCIES TO TAKE OFFENSE, BECOME HOSTILE, AND THEN HOLD GRUDGES USUALLY ARE NOTABLE (I-Do EXCEEDS I-De BY A T-SCORE DIFFERENCE OF 15 OR MORE POINTS, AND HOS IS T65 OR ABOVE AND/OR TSC/R IS T70 OR ABOVE), WRITE:

Respondent possesses the cardinal characteristics of the paranoid personality disorder.

C. Narcissistic Personality Disorder

(1) IF THE NARCISSISTIC SUPPLEMENTARY ITEM SET (Table 5.4) IS AT LEVEL III OR ABOVE AND (2) AN INFLATED SENSE OF SELF IMPORTANCE AND BEING SPECIAL RESULTS IN EXAGGERATEDLY POSITIVE SELF PRESENTATION AND SOCIAL BOLDNESS IN THE ABSENCE OF A CHEERFUL, EXTROVERTED OUTLOOK (ME IS T45 OR BELOW WITH SYMPTOMATIC SPECIAL SCALES GENERALLY LOW; 8CON IS T45 OR BELOW; 2PR IS T45 OR BELOW; THE SUM OF T-SCORES FOR 3DSA, 4SI AND 9IMP USUALLY IS ABOVE 170, AND SOC AND TSC/I ARE T47 OR BELOW, BUT HYP IS T55 OR BELOW) AND (3) EMPATHIC CAPACITY AND INTERPERSONAL SENSITIVITY USUALLY ARE LACKING (3NA AND 6N ARE T52 OR BELOW, AND 6P IS T56 OR BELOW) AND (4) EXPLOITATIVE ATTITUDE USUALLY IS PRESENT (I-Do IS IN THE RANGE T60–69 OR, WHATEVER ITS LEVEL, IS AT LEAST 15 T-SCORE POINTS ABOVE I-De), WRITE:

Respondent possesses the cardinal characteristics of the narcissistic personality disorder.

D. Histrionic Personality Disorder

(1) IF THE HISTRIONIC SUPPLEMENTARY ITEMS SET (Table 5.4) IS AT LEVEL III OR ABOVE AND (2) THE NEED TO BE THE CENTER OF ATTENTION RESULTS IN THE SAME PATTERN AND LEVELS AS FOR THE NARCISSISTIC PERSONALITY SCALE LISTING AND (3) EMPATHIC CAPACITY AND INTERPERSONAL SENSITIVITY ARE COMPARABLE TO THOSE OF THE NARCISSISTIC PERSONALITY DISORDER AND (4) THERE FREQUENTLY IS A READINESS TO USE OTHERS IN ORDER TO MEET DEPENDENCY NEEDS (I-Do IS T70 OR ABOVE, AND I-De MAY ALSO BE AS HIGH AS T60) AND (5) SEDUCTIVE AND PROVOCATIVE BEHAVIOR FREQUENTLY LEADS TO SEXUAL DIFFICULTIES (I-SP IS T70 OR ABOVE, AND, FOR MALES Pe IS T65 OR ABOVE; INSPECT RELEVANT ITEMS) AND (6) OFTEN AN IMPRESSIONISTIC COGNITIVE STYLE LEADS TO RESPONSE INCONSISTENCIES THAT CANNOT BE ACCOUNTED FOR BY POOR READING COMPREHENSION OR MENTAL CONFUSION (TR + CLS IS 6 OR 7), WRITE:

Respondent possesses the cardinal characteristics of the histrionic personality disorder.

E. Borderline Personality Disorder

(1) IF THE BORDERLINE SUPPLEMENTARY ITEM SET (Table 5.4) IS AT LEVEL III OR ABOVE AND (2) WIDELY VARIED SYMPTOMS SIGNAL DISTRESS (ME EXCEEDS T70, AND THESE SPECIAL SCALES ELEVATE: EITHER DEP OR TSC/D EQUALS T65–69 AND THE OTHER IS T60–64; MOR AND/OR I-SC ARE T65–69; 8COG AND 2MD ARE T60–65; TSC/T IS T60–69; HOS IS T61–65 AND TSC/R IS T60 OR ABOVE) AND (3) DURING CRISES, WHOSE REOCCURRING PRESENCE IS A HALLMARK OF THIS PERSONALITY DISORDER, THE FOREGOING GENERALLY INCREASE, AND OTHER SEVERE SYMPTOMS APPEAR (S+ IS T59 OR ABOVE AND/OR I-DS IS T65 OR ABOVE) AND (4) INTENSE INTERPERSONAL RELATIONS ARE PURSUED IN THE FACE OF EXQUISITE HYPERSEN-SITIVITY AND SOCIAL ANXIETY (THE SUM OF 3DSA, 4SI, AND 9IMP IS 120–129 AND 6P IS T65 OR ABOVE, BUT SOC AND TSC/I ARE AROUND T50) AND (5) IMPULSIVITY IS ELEVATED, INCREASING WITH CRISES (SEE 3 ABOVE), AND FREQUENTLY IS ACCOMPANIED BY SUBSTANCE ABUSE (HYP AND 9PMA ARE T59 OR ABOVE AND AMac IS T65 OR ABOVE) AND (6) DURING SERIOUS DEPRESSION, SUI-

CIDAL THOUGHTS AND BEHAVIORS ARE NOTABLE (TSC/D OR DEP IS T70 OR ABOVE WHILE THE OTHER IS T65–69, AND 2PR IS T55 OR BELOW AND SUICIDAL INDICATORS ARE PRESENT) AND (7) UNSTA-BLE SELF IMAGE SOMETIMES INVOLVES GENDER CONFUSION (I-SP IS T70; AND FOR MALES Pe IS T70; AND FOR FEMALES FEM IS EITHER T70 OR ABOVE OR BELOW T40 OR T35 FOR RESPONDENTS WITH 14 OR MORE YEARS OF FORMAL EDUCATION), WRITE:

Respondent has the cardinal characteristics of the borderline personality disorder.

F. Passive Aggressive Personality Disorder

(1) IF THE PASSIVE AGGRESSIVE SUPPLEMENTARY ITEM SET (Table 5.4) IS AT LEVEL III OR ABOVE AND (2) THE PERSON FEELS POWER-LESS, EXTERNALLY CONTROLLED AND UNABLE TO RESOLVE THIS DILEMMA BY PERSONAL EFFORT (I-De EXCEEDS I-Do BY 15 OR MORE T-SCORE POINTS; E/Cy IS T65 OR ABOVE BUT FREQUENTLY WITH Ho AND TSC/S NOT QUITE REACHING THIS LEVEL; 8CON IS T65 OR ABOVE) AND (3) OPPOSITIONAL ATTITUDES APPEAR ALONG WITH RESTLESS IMPULSIVITY (TSC/R IS T70 OR ABOVE AND EXCEEDS HOS WHICH IS AROUND T55; AUT IS T65 OR ABOVE AND EXCEEDS 4AC WHICH IS T55 OR BELOW; AND EITHER 9PMA AND/OR HYP IS T60 OR ABOVE) AND (4) ANXIETY OVER RETALIATION FOR (3) IS PRESENT PLUS FEELINGS OF SOCIAL AWKWARDNESS, DISCOMFORT AND VULNERABILITY (TSC/T IS T58–65; THE T-SCORE SUM OF 3DSA, 4SI AND 9IMP IS 130–140, AND SOC AND TSC/I ARE T58–65; 6P IS T60 OR ABOVE) AND (5) THE PERSON SUFFERS FROM POOR SELF IMAGE BUT WITHOUT DEPRESSION (MOR AND/OR I-SC ARE T65–69; 2MD IS T60–65; ME IS T58–65; TSC/D AND DEP ARE OFTEN T58 OR BELOW, AND THEY ARE LOWER THAN MOR AND/OR I-SC) AND (6) HE/SHE FEELS ALIENATED, AND DEPRIVED OF DESIRED FAMILY SUPPORT (EITHER 4SOA OR 8SOA IS T60–69 AND THE OTHER IS T65 OR ABOVE; FAM IS T60 OR ABOVE AND 4FD IS T65 OR ABOVE), WRITE:

This individual possesses the cardinal characteristics of the passive aggressive personality disorder.

G. Dependent Personality Disorder

(1) IF THE DEPENDENT PERSONALITY DISORDER ITEM SET (Table 5.4) IS LEVEL III OR ABOVE AND (2) THE DEPENDENCY TRAIT IS PRE-EMINENT (I-De IS T60 OR ABOVE AND USUALLY 20 OR MORE T-SCORE POINTS ABOVE I-Do; Astvn IS T45 OR BELOW FOR FEMALES) AND (3) HE/SHE IS EMOTIONALLY UNABLE TO CHALLENGE AUTHORITY OR

TO EXPRESS HOSTILITY OPENLY (AUT AND 4AC ARE T49 OR BELOW; HOS IS T44 OR BELOW, AND TSC/R IS OFTEN AT THIS LEVEL BUT SOMETIMES IS T58 OR ABOVE) AND (4) POOR SELF IMAGE IS AC-COMPANIED BY FEELINGS OF INADEQUACY (MOR AND I-SC ARE T65 OR ABOVE; 2MD AND 8COG ARE T65 OR ABOVE) AND (5) HE/SHE SEEKS SAFETY IN CONVENTIONAL AND OVERLY TRUSTING ATTI-TUDES, YET CONTINUES TO FEEL SOCIALLY VULNERABLE (5C IS T60 OR ABOVE; E/Cy, Ho, TSC/S ARE T45 OR BELOW; 6P IS T60 OR ABOVE) AND (6) ANERGIA AND A DEFECT OF INITIATIVE ARE NOTABLE (9PMA AND HYP ARE T47 OR BELOW, AND 2PR IS T59 OR ABOVE; 8CON IS T65 OR ABOVE) AND (7) HE/SHE USUALLY IS SOMEWHAT EMOTIONALLY DISTRAUGHT OVER MEETING DEPENDENCY NEEDS (TSC/D AND DEP ARE T60 OR ABOVE AND/OR TSC/T IS T58–65), WRITE:

This person has the cardinal characteristics of the dependent personality disorder.

H. Obsessive-Compulsive Personality Disorder

(1) IF THE OBSESSIVE-COMPULSIVE SUPPLEMENTARY ITEM SET (Table 5.4) IS LEVEL III OR ABOVE, USUALLY WITHOUT RITUAL COMPUL-SIONS (I-OC NOT ABOVE T60) AND (2) A CONFORMING, MORAL OUT-LOOK IS FOREMOST IN IMPORTANCE (5C IS USUALLY T70 OR ABOVE; THE SUM OF T-SCORES FOR 3NA AND 6N IS 125 OR ABOVE WITH ONE POSSIBLY T70, AND 9AMO IS T45 OR BELOW) AND (3) SELF RESTRAINT AND DRIVE CONTROL ARE OVERVALUED, AND EMOTIONAL INVUL-NERABILITY IS A PERCEIVED URGENT NEED (I-Do IS T60–69 AND/OR 15 POINTS ABOVE I-De; 9PMA IS T41 OR BELOW AND HYP IS T47 OR BELOW; 8CON IS T45 OR BELOW; 6P IS T50 OR BELOW) AND (4) EXPRESSIONS OF SYMPTOMS/PROBLEMS ARE SYSTEMATICALLY DE-NIED, PARTICULARLY FOR ALL FORMS OF HOSTILITY OR CONFLICT AND FOR SHORTCOMINGS IN SOCIAL CONTEXTS (ME IS T40 OR BELOW; HOS IS T40 OR BELOW AND TSC/R IS T47 OR BELOW; Ho, E/Cy, AND TSC/S ARE TYPICALLY T45 AND BELOW; AUT AND 4AC ARE T49 OR BELOW; 4SOA AND 8SOA ARE T47 OR BELOW; THE T-SCORE SUM OF 3DSA, 4SI, AND 9IMP IS 170 OR ABOVE AND SOC AND TSC/I ARE T52 OR BELOW) AND (5) AN EXCEPTION TO (4) IS THAT SOMATIC COM-PLAINTS ARE SOMETIMES ADMITTED (TSC/B AND HEA MAY BE T60 OR ABOVE) AND (6) DURING CRISES, THE RIGID DEFENSES NOTED IN (3 AND 2) CAN LEAD TO OVERCONTROLLED HOSTILITY, AUTHORITY CONFLICT, AND ANXIETY (OH IS T60 OR ABOVE; AUT AND 4AC ARE T60 OR ABOVE; TSC/T IS T60–69), WRITE:

Respondent possesses the cardinal characteristics of the obsessive-compulsive personality disorder.

I. Avoidant Personality Disorder

(1) IF THE AVOIDANT SUPPLEMENTARY ITEM SET (Table 5.4) IS AT LEVEL III OR ABOVE, ALONG WITH LEVEL III ELEVATIONS FOR THE AVOIDANT-SCHIZOTYPAL-SCHIZOID AND AVOIDANT-SCHIZOTYPAL CORE ITEM SETS AND (2) SOCIAL INADEQUACY, ANXIETY, WITHDRAWAL AND VULNERABILITY ARE UNBOUNDED (THE T-SCORE SUM OF 3DSA, 4SI, AND 9IMP IS LESS THAN 120, AND SOC AND TSC/I ARE T70 OR ABOVE; 6P IS T65 OR MORE) AND (3) THE INDIVIDUAL FEELS IMMOBILIZED (8CON IS T69 OR ABOVE; 2PR IS T65 OR ABOVE) AND (4) HE/SHE HAS A VERY POOR SELF CONCEPT AND STRONG FEELINGS OF INFERIORITY AND EMBARRASSMENT (MOR AND/OR I-SC ARE T70 OR ABOVE; 8COG AND 2MD ARE T70 OR ABOVE) AND (5) SYMPTOM EXPRESSION IS EXCEEDINGLY HIGH, WITH PARTICULAR EMPHASIS ON EMOTIONAL ELEMENTS THAT ACCOMPANY THE TRAITS LISTED IN (3 AND 2), BUT WITHOUT PSYCHOTIC ELEVATIONS (ME OFTEN IS T70 OR ABOVE; TSC/D AND DEP ARE T65 OR ABOVE; TSC/T IS T60–69; PSY, 8BSE, I-RD USUALLY ARE BELOW T60) AND (6) DUE TO WITHDRAWAL, EXPRESSIONS OF ALIENATION, FAMILY CONFLICT, AND HOSTILITY ARE FREQUENTLY MILD (4SOA AND 8SOA ARE T56–64; FAM AND 4AC ARE T57–63; HOS AND TSC/R ARE T58–63), WRITE:

Respondent possesses the cardinal characteristics of the avoidant personality disorder.

J. Schizotypal Personality Disorder

(1) THE SCHIZOTYPAL SUPPLEMENTARY ITEM SET (Table 5.4) IS AT LEVEL III OR ABOVE, AND THE AVOIDANT-SCHIZOTYPAL-SCHIZOID AND AVOIDANT-SCHIZOTYPAL CORE ITEM SETS ARE LEVEL III OR ABOVE AND (2) SOCIAL INADEQUACY, ANXIETY, WITHDRAWAL, AND VULNERABILITY ARE EXTREME (THE T-SCORE SUM OF 3DSA, 4SI, AND 9IMP IS 120–129, AND SOC AND TSC/I ARE T60–69; 6P IS T65 OR ABOVE) AND (3) HE/SHE HAS A POOR SELF CONCEPT AND STRONG FEELINGS OF INADEQUACY (MOR AND/OR I-SC ARE T70 OR ABOVE; 8COG AND 2MD ARE T65 OR ABOVE) AND (4) SYMPTOM EXPRESSION IS EXCEEDINGLY HIGH, WITH PSYCHOTIC INDICATORS ELEVATED ALONG WITH EMOTIONAL DISTRESS AND FEELINGS OF BEING TOO TROUBLED TO WORK OUT PROBLEMS (ME IS T70 OR ABOVE; PSY, I-RD, 8BSE, ORG, I-DS AND/OR S+ ARE T65 OR ABOVE; TSC/D AND DEP ARE T65–69; TSC/T IS T60–69; 8CON IS T65 OR ABOVE) AND (5) DUE TO WITHDRAWAL, EXPRESSIONS OF ALIENATION AND HOSTILITY ARE FREQUENTLY MILD (4SOA AND 8SOA ARE T56–64; HOS AND TSC/R ARE T58–63), WRITE:

Respondent possesses the cardinal characteristics of the schizotypal personality disorder.

K. Schizoid Personality Disorder

(1) IF THE AVOIDANT-SCHIZOTYPAL-SCHIZOID SUPPLEMENTARY ITEM SET (Table 5.4) IS AT LEVEL III OR ABOVE, WHILE THE AVOIDANT-SCHIZOTYPAL SUPPLEMENTARY ITEM SET IS AT LEVEL I OR BELOW AND (2) NEITHER THE AVOIDANT NOR SCHIZOTYPAL SUPPLEMENTARY ITEM SET IS AT LEVEL III OR ABOVE AND (3) SOCIAL INADEQUACY, ANXIETY, AND WITHDRAWAL ARE PROMINENT, BUT WITHOUT FEELINGS OF SOCIAL VULNERABILITY (THE T-SCORE SUM OF 3DSA, 4SI, AND 9IMP IS 120–129, AND SOC AND TSC/I ARE T70 OR ABOVE; 6P IS AROUND T50) AND (4) THE INDIVIDUAL IS ANERGIC, HAS A DEFECT OF INITIATIVE, AVOIDS STIMULATION, AND IS ANHEDONIC BUT WITHOUT SIGNS OF DEPRESSION (2PR IS T65 OR ABOVE; 8CON IS T65 OR ABOVE; 9PMA AND HYP ARE T47 OR BELOW; DEP AND TSC/D ARE T55 OR BELOW) AND (5) THE QUITE VARIED SYMPTOM INDICATORS SEEN IN AVOIDANTS AND SCHIZOTYPALS ARE ABSENT (ME IS T56 OR BELOW) AND (6) SOCIAL DISCONNECTEDNESS IS EVIDENCED BY ABSENCE OF CONCERN OVER SOCIAL ISOLATION (4SOA AND 8SOA ARE BELOW T55; FAM AND 4AC ARE AROUND T50) AND (7) DRUG ABUSE IS OFTEN PRESENT, WRITE:

Respondent possesses the cardinal characteristics of the schizoid personality disorder.

L. Atypical or Mixed Personality Disorder

(1) IF EITHER NONE OF THE FOREGOING PERSONALITY DISORDER STATEMENTS HAS BEEN WRITTEN OR A STATEMENT HAS BEEN WRITTEN, BUT WITHOUT BEING DEPENDENT ON THE FOLLOWING ADDITIONAL LINES OF EVIDENCE AND (2) TWO OR MORE OF THE REMAINING SUPPLEMENTARY ITEM SETS IS AT LEVEL II OR ABOVE AND (3) OTHER SUPPLEMENTARY ITEM SETS MAY OR MAY NOT BE AT LEVEL I AND (4) OTHER SPECIAL SCALE INDICATORS ARE PRESENT THAT ARE NOT LIKELY THE CONSEQUENCE OF AN AXIS I CONDITION OR OF ANY OTHER PERSONALITY DISORDER FOR WHICH A STATEMENT WAS WRITTEN, WRITE:

Respondent has a mixed (or atypical) personality disorder.

IF THERE IS A MIXED PERSONALITY DISORDER, INCLUDE IN THE PRECEDING STATEMENT FURTHER DESCRIPTORS THAT CHARACTERIZE THE NATURE OF THE DISORDER IN TERMS OF THE SPECIAL SCALES AND SUPPLEMENTARY ITEM SETS USED TO REACH THE CONCLUSION. IF THE PERSONALITY DISORDER IS TOO COMPLEX OR OBSCURE TO CHARACTERIZE SUCCINCTLY IN THIS MANNER, THEN IN THE PRECEDING STATEMENT, SUBSTITUTE THE WORD *atypical* FOR THE WORD *mixed*.

M. Further Distinctions for Identifying Personality Disorders

(1) IF A SUPPLEMENTARY ITEM SET IS AT LEVEL II AND (2) THE APPLICABLE SPECIAL SCALE INDICATORS ARE CLEARLY PRESENT (Table 5.3) AND (3) COMPETING SPECIAL SCALE AND/OR SUPPLEMENTARY ITEM SET INDICATORS ARE ESSENTIALLY ABSENT, WRITE:

This is probably a _____ personality disorder. COMPLETE THE STATEMENT BY ADAPTING A PERSONALITY STATEMENT FROM *A* THROUGH *K*.

(1) IF EVERYTHING IS AS STATED IN THE PRECEDING, (2) EXCEPT THAT THE SUPPLEMENTARY ITEM SET IS AT LEVEL I, OR (3) IF A PATTERN OF SPECIAL SCALE ELEVATIONS CLOSELY RESEMBLES ONE OF THE SPECIFIC PERSONALITY DISORDERS BUT WITHOUT THE CORRESPONDING SUPPLEMENTARY ITEM SET BEING AT LEAST AT LEVEL I, WRITE:

There is no evidence of a personality disorder but a personality type is indicated.

(1) IF A SUPPLEMENTARY ITEM SET IS AT LEVEL I OR ABOVE AND (2) IS NOT SUPPORTED BY SUBSTANTIAL EVIDENCE BASED ON THE RELEVANT SPECIAL SCALES, DO NOT WRITE A SPECIFIC PERSONALITY DISORDER STATEMENT. INSTEAD CONSIDER WHETHER THE EVIDENCE POINTS TO A MIXED OR ATYPICAL PERSONALITY DISORDER.

V. INCONSISTENT OR CONFLICTUAL RESPONDING

A. Morality and Virtue

IF THE T-SCORES FOR 3NA AND 6N TOTAL TO AT LEAST 125 AND 9AMO IS AT LEAST T62, WRITE:

Respondent appears to have a conflict over moral values. He/She seems to be unable to decide whether honesty and friendliness, or selfishness and opportunism, constitute the desirable lifestyle.

IF RESPONDENT IS A FEMALE AND A STATEMENT HAS BEEN WRITTEN FOR I-SP, ADD:

Respondent's conflict may involve impulses to act out sexually.

(IF RESPONDENT IS MARRIED, SUBSTITUTE "extramaritally" FOR "sexually.")

B. Social Anxiety

IF A STATEMENT HAS BEEN WRITTEN IN THE Social Adjustment SECTION THAT REFLECTS SOCIAL ANXIETY AND/OR AVOIDANT TENDENCY (i.e., 3DSA, 4SI, 9IMP) AND 9PMA IS ELEVATED (SEE SECTION ON Extraversion), WRITE:

Respondent's shyness and reticence may be causing difficulty in satisfying his/her need for social stimulation. Such a conflict can be a source of emotional symptoms.

C. Anxiety and Depression

IF NONE OF THE ANXIETY SCALES HAS WARRANTED A STATEMENT BUT THE RESPONDENT HAS ENDORSED AT LEAST TWO OF THE FOLLOWING ITEMS:

I feel anxiety about something or someone almost all the time. (337)
Almost every day something happens to frighten me. (360)
I worry quite a bit over possible misfortunes. (431)
Several times a week I feel as if something dreadful is about to happen. (543)

WRITE:

Respondent does not have high trait anxiety but for some reason regards himself/herself as an anxious person. This discrepancy should be investigated.

IF NONE OF THE DEPRESSION SCALES HAS WARRANTED A STATEMENT BUT RESPONDENT HAS ENDORSED AT LEAST TWO OF THE FOLLOWING ITEMS:

I believe my sins are unpardonable. (209)
Most of the time I wish I were dead. (339)
I deserve severe punishment for my sins. (413)
The future seems hopeless to me. (526)

WRITE:

Respondent does not appear to be clinically depressed but may wish to create such an impression. This possibility should be investigated.

VI. PROGNOSIS WITH THERAPY

A. Psychotherapy

With psychotherapy, counseling or other "talking therapies" that require active cooperation by the patient as opposed to regimens of medication, the following observations should prove useful.

A number of scales can be involved in making prognostic statements concerning patients. These include the social maladjustment, suspiciousness, distrust, and authority conflict scales. High scores lead to a statement of poor prognosis, for reasons inherent in the characteristics measured by these scales: The rules follow:

IF THE SUM OF 3DSA + 4SI + 9IMP IS LESS THAN 120, WRITE:

The prognosis with forms of psychotherapy requiring active cooperation by the patient is poor because this patient is too socially anxious to be able to form a therapeutic alliance with a health care delivery person.

IF EITHER 4AC OR AUT IS GREATER THAN T70, WRITE:

The prognosis with forms of psychotherapy requiring active cooperation by the patient is poor because of this patient's hostile attitude toward authority figures.

IF TSC/S IS GREATER THAN T65, AND/OR IF S+ IS T60 OR ABOVE, WRITE:

The prognosis with forms of psychotherapy requiring active cooperation by the patient is poor because this patient characteristically distrusts the motives of others and will thus be unable to form a therapeutic alliance with a health care delivery person.

IF 8CON IS T70 OR ABOVE AND ANY OF THE PRECEDING STATE-MENTS HAS BEEN WRITTEN, ADD TO THE STATEMENT:

This patient also appears to lack sufficient motivation for self-improvement.

IF 8CON IS T70 OR ABOVE AND NONE OF THE PRECEDING STATE-MENTS HAS BEEN WRITTEN, WRITE:

The prognosis for this patient is guarded because he/she appears to lack sufficient motivation for self-improvement.

IF NONE OF THE PRECEDING STATEMENTS HAS BEEN WRITTEN, WRITE:

The prognosis for this patient with forms of psychotherapy requiring active cooperation by the patient is favorable.

B. Hospitalization

In some cases, a prognostic issue may be whether the patient needs to be hospitalized, for example, patients for whom a statement has been written under Suicidal Tendency (II; A; 2). Scores on two other scales are relevant here.

IF WA IS IN THE RANGE T60–69, WRITE:

Patient complains that his/her daily life functioning is impaired but not sufficiently to require hospitalization.

IF WA IS T70 OR ABOVE, WRITE:

Patient feels that he/she is totally unable to function productively in his/her normal circumstances. A period of hospitalization is indicated.

IF A PATIENT IS SERIOUSLY DISTURBED ACCORDING TO SYMPTOM SCALES AND Cn IS ABOVE T65, WRITE:

Despite his/her serious psychopathology, he/she does not require hospitalization.

SPECIAL NOTES

1. If the respondent is African-American, add T5 to statements under:
   HOS

> TSC/R
> OH
> TSC/S
> S+

2. If the respondent is African-American, add T10 to the statement under 9AMO.

3. If the respondent is Hispanic-American, add T5 to statements under:

AUT	3NA
DEP	6PI
HOS	6N
MOR	8SOA
ORG	8COG
PHO	8CON
PSY	8BSE

4. Sources for the modifications in Special Notes 1–3: Gynther (1972); Hutton, Miner, Blades, & Langfeldt (1992); Montgomery, Arnold, & Orozco (1990).

5. All item numbers cited in this appendix are for the original booklet MMPI group form. Form R item numbers are given after the diagonal slash whenever the Form R sequence differs from the original group form.

APPENDIX VI
SPECIAL SCALES
EXCLUDED FROM
APPENDIX V

With the exception of OH, Ho, AMac and the Wiggins scales, none of the scales discussed in this book and recommended for clinical use has a firm basis in experimental investigation. Rather, the evaluation of these scales has been based on their clinical use with thousands of respondents, as we noted in Chapter 1.

Over the years, a number of other special scales were scored in the computer program at the Indiana University Medical Center and were eventually discarded as not clinically useful. The Harris and Lingoes scales that fell into this class are identified in Table 3.2. We discussed the shortcomings of so-called ego-strength scales in Chapter 5. Scales like Welsh's A and R Factors are relatively insensitive because of multidimensionality. A few scales, like Navran's Dependency scale and some of the Pepper and Strong scales, were discarded because much superior special scales are available. Most of the scales that we do not recommend for clinical use simply did not appear to measure an identifiable meaningful characteristic or condition. With rare exceptions like A, R and Es, most of the scales we discarded had never been subjected to independent experimental scrutiny. And none—including A, R and Es—has any sound research support.

We acknowledge that other clinicians may have found some of the scales in this appendix to be useful. Assessment styles vary; there is no absolute method for dealing clinically with special scales. In contexts different from our testing grounds, some of the scales in this appendix may be helpful to the clinician.

A Factor (Welsh, 1956)
Admission of Symptoms (Little & Fisher, 1958)

159

Alcoholism (Rosenberg, 1972)
Anxiety Index (Welsh, 1952)
Autism (Stein, 1968)
Caudality (Williams, 1952)
Denial of Symptoms (Little & Fisher, 1958)
Dependency (Navran, 1954)
Dominance (Gough, McCloskey, & Meehl, 1951)
Dominance, revised (Gough, 1957)
Ego-Control (Block, 1965)
Ego-Resilience (Block, 1965)
Ego-Strength (Barron, 1953)
Electroshock Prognosis (Feldman, 1951)
Extraversion (Giedt & Downing, 1961)
Facilitation-Inhibition (Ullman, 1962)
Factors I–III (Eichman, 1961–62)
Homosexuality (Panton, 1959)
Index of Psychopathology (Sines & Silver, 1963)
Internalization Ratio (Welsh, 1952)
Low Back Pain (Hanvik, 1951)
Manifest Anxiety (Taylor, 1953)
Neuroticism (Winne, 1951)
Obvious–Subtle Scales (except Depression–Subtle) (Wiener & Harmon, 1946)
Pepper & Strong Scales (except Altruism) (Pepper & Strong, 1958)
Pharisaic Virtue (Cook & Medley, 1954)
Prejudice (Gough, 1951)
R Factor (Welsh, 1956)
Role-Playing (McClelland, 1951)
Rosen Scales (Rosen, 1962)
Self-Sufficiency (Wolff, 1955)
Six Signs (Peterson, 1954)
Social Responsibility (Gough, McCloskey, & Meehl, 1952)
Social Status (Gough, 1948)
Test-Taking Defensiveness (Hanley, 1957)

REFERENCES

Adams, H. B., & Cooper, G. D. (1962). Three measures of ego strength and prognosis for psychotherapy. *Journal of Clinical Psychology, 18,* 490–494.

Adams, H. B., Cooper, G. D., & Carrera, R. N. (1963). The Rorschach and the MMPI: A concurrent validity study. *Journal of Projective Techniques, 27,* 23–24.

Affleck, D. C., & Garfield, S. L. (1960). The prediction of psychosis with the MMPI. *Journal of Clinical Psychology, 16,* 24–26.

American Psychiatric Association. (1952). *Diagnostic and statistical manual: Mental disorders.* Washington, DC: Author.

American Psychiatric Association. (1980). *Diagnostic and statistical manual of mental disorders (3rd ed.).* Washington, DC: Author.

American Psychiatric Association. (1987). *Diagnostic and statistical manual of mental disorders (3rd ed., rev.)* (III-R). Washington, DC: Author.

American Psychiatric Association. (1993). *DSM-IV draft criteria. Task Force on DSM-IV.* Washington, DC: Author.

American Psychiatric Association. (1994). *Diagnostic and statistical manual of mental disorders (4th ed.).* Washington, DC: Author.

Apfeldorf, M., & Hunley, P. J. (1975). Application of MMPI alcoholism scales to older alcoholics and problem drinkers. *Journal of Studies on Alcohol, 36,* 645–653.

Archer, R. P. (1987). *Using the MMPI with adolescents.* Hillsdale, NJ: Lawrence Erlbaum Associates.

Archer, R. P., & Krishnamurthy, R. (1993a). Combining the Rorschach and the MMPI in the assessment of adolescents. *Journal of Personality Assessment, 60,* 132–140.

Archer, R. P., & Krishnamurthy, R. (1993b). A review of MMPI and Rorschach interrelationships in adult samples. *Journal of Personality Assessment, 61,* 277–293.

Ardell, D. B. (1977). *High level wellness.* Emmaus, PA: Rodale Press.

Ashton, S. G., & Goldberg, L. R. (1973). In response to Jackson's challenge: The comparative validity of personality scales constructed by the external (empirical) strategy and scales developed intuitively by experts, novices, and laymen. *Journal of Research in Personality, 7*, 1–20.

Barefoot, J. C., Dahlstrom, W. G., & Williams, R. B., Jr. (1983). Hostility, CHD incidence, and total mentality: A 25-year follow-up study of 255 physicians. *Psychosomatic Medicine, 45*, 59–63.

Barger, P. M., & Sechrest, L. B. (1961). Convergent and discriminant validity of four Holtzman Inkblot Test variables. *Journal of Psychological Studies, 12*, 227–236.

Barron, F. (1953). An ego-strength scale which predicts response to psychotherapy. *Journal of Consulting Psychology, 17*, 327–333.

Beck, S. J. (1952). *Rorschach's test: III. Advances in interpretation.* New York: Grune & Stratton.

Beck, S. J., Rabin, A. I., Thiesen, W. G., Molish, H. B., & Thetford, W. N. (1950). The normal personality as projected in the Rorschach test. *Journal of Psychology, 30*, 241–298.

Ben-Porath, Y. S., & Butcher, J. N. (1989). Psychometric stability of rewritten MMPI items. *Journal of Personality Assessment, 53*, 645–653.

Ben-Porath, Y. S., Butcher, J. N., & Graham, J. R. (1991). Contribution of the MMPI-2 content scales to the differential diagnosis of schizophrenia and major depression. *Psychological Assessment, 3*, 634–640.

Ben-Porath, Y. S., McCully, E., & Almagor, M. (1993). Incremental validity of the MMPI-2 content scales in the assessment of personality and psychopathology by self-report. *Journal of Personality Assessment, 61*, 557–575.

Blackburn, R. (1968). Personality in relation to extreme aggression in psychiatric offenders. *British Journal of Psychiatry, 114*, 821–828.

Blackburn, R. (1972). Dimensions of hostility and aggression in abnormal offenders. *Journal of Consulting & Clinical Psychology, 21*, 282–283.

Block, J. (1965). *The challenge of response sets.* New York: Appleton-Century-Crofts.

Boerger, A. R. (1975). *The utility of some alternative approaches to MMPI scale construction.* Unpublished doctoral dissertation, Kent State University, Kent, OH.

Bond, J. A. (1986). Inconsistent responding to repeated MMPI items: Is its major cause really carelessness? *Journal of Personality Assessment, 50*, 50–64.

Brems, C., & Johnson, M. E. (1990). Further explorations of the Egocentricity Index in an inpatient psychiatric population. *Journal of Clinical Psychology, 46*, 675–679.

Buechley, R., & Ball, H. (1952). A new test of "validity" for the group MMPI. *Journal of Consulting Psychology, 16*, 299–301.

Burke, H., & Marcus, R. (1977). MacAndrew MMPI Alcoholism scale: Alcoholism and drug addictiveness. *Journal of Psychology, 96*, 141–148.

Burkhart, B. R., Christian, W. L., & Gynther, M. D. (1978). Item subtlety and faking on the MMPI: A paradoxical relationship. *Journal of Personality Assessment, 42*, 76–80.

Buss, A. H., & Durkee, A. (1957). An inventory for assessing different kinds of hostility. *Journal of Consulting Psychology, 21*, 343–349.

Butcher, J. N. (1978). *Minnesota Multiphasic Personality Inventory: Computerized scoring and interpreting services.* In O. K. Buros (Ed.), *The eighth mental measurements yearbook* (pp. 942–945). Highland Park, NJ: Gryphon Press.

Butcher, J. N. (1990). *The MMPI-2 in psychological treatment.* New York: Oxford University Press.

Butcher, J. N. (1994). Psychological assessment of airline pilot applicants with the MMPI-2. *Journal of Personality Assessment, 62*, 31–44.

Butcher, J. N., Dahlstrom, W. G., Graham, J. R., Tellegen, A., & Kaemmer, B. (1989). *Minnesota Multiphasic Personality Inventory (MMPI-2). Manual for administration and scoring.* Minneapolis: University of Minnesota Press.

Butcher, J. N., Graham, J. R., Williams, C. L., & Ben-Porath, Y. S. (1990). *Development and use of the MMPI-2 content scales.* Minneapolis: University of Minnesota Press.

Butcher, J. N., & Tellegen, A. (1978). Common methodological problems in MMPI research. *Journal of Consulting Psychology, 46*, 620–628.

Calvin, J. (1975). *A replicated study of the concurrent validity of the Harris subscales for the MMPI.* Unpublished doctoral dissertation, Kent State University, Kent, OH.

Cernovsky, Z. (1986). Masculinity-femininity scale of the MMPI and intellectual functioning of female addicts. *Journal of Clinical Psychology, 42,* 310–312.

Chojnacki, J. T., & Walsh, W. B. (1994). The consistency of scores between the Harris-Lingoes Subscales of the MMPI and MMPI-2. *Journal of Personality Assessment, 62,* 157–165.

Christian, W. L., Burkhart, B. R., & Gynther, M. D. (1978). Subtle-obvious ratings of MMPI items: New interest in an old concept. *Journal of Clinical Psychology, 46,* 1178–1186.

Clopton, J. R. (1979a). Development of special MMPI scales. In C. S. Newmark (Ed.), *MMPI clinical and research trends.* New York: Praeger.

Clopton, J. R. (1979b). MMPI and suicide. In C. S. Newmark (Ed.), *MMPI clinical and research trends.* New York: Praeger.

Clopton, J. R., & Neuringer, C. (1979). MMPI cannot say scores: Normative data and degree of profile distortion. *Journal of Personality Assessment, 41,* 511–513.

Colligan, R. C., Osborne, D., Swenson, W. M., & Offord, K. P. (1983). *The MMPI: A contemporary normative study.* New York: Praeger.

Colligan, R. C., Osborne, D., Swenson, W. M., & Offord, K. P. (1989). *The MMPI: A contemporary normative study of adults* (2nd ed.). Odessa, FL: Psychological Assessment Resources.

Cook, W. W., & Medley, D. M. (1954). Proposed hostility and Pharisaic-virtue scales for the MMPI. *Journal of Applied Psychology, 38,* 414–418.

Costa, P. T., Jr., Zonderman, A. B., McCrae, R. R., & Williams, R. B., Jr. (1985). Content and comprehensiveness in the MMPI: An item factor analysis in a normal adult sample. *Journal of Personality & Social Psychology, 48,* 925–933.

Cronbach, L. J. (1951). Coefficient alpha and the internal structure of tests. *Psychometrika, 16,* 297–334.

Crumpton, E., Cantor, J. M., & Batiste, C. (1960). A factor analytic study of Barron's Ego-Strength scale. *Journal of Clinical Psychology, 16,* 283–291.

Cuadra, C. A. (1956). A scale for control in psychological adjustment. In G. S. Welsh & W. G. Dahlstrom (Eds.), *Basic readings on the MMPI in psychology and medicine* (pp. 235–254). Minneapolis, MN: University of Minnesota Press.

Dahlstrom, W. G. (1969). Recurrent issues in the development of the MMPI. In J. N. Butcher (Ed.), *MMPI: Research developments and clinical applications.* New York: McGraw-Hill.

Dahlstrom, W. G., & Welsh, G. S. (1960). *An MMPI handbook: A Guide to use in clinical practice and research.* Minneapolis, MN: University of Minnesota Press.

Dahlstrom, W. G., Welsh, G. S., & Dahlstrom, L. E. (1972). *An MMPI handbook: Vol. I. Clinical interpretation* (rev. ed.). Minneapolis, MN: University of Minnesota Press.

Dahlstrom, W. G., Welsh, G. S., & Dahlstrom, L. E. (1975). *An MMPI handbook: Vol. II. Research applications* (rev. ed.). Minneapolis, MN: University of Minnesota Press.

deGroot, G. W., & Adamson, J. D. (1973). Responses of psychiatric inpatients to the MacAndrew Alcoholism scale. *Quarterly Journal of Studies on Alcohol, 34,* 1133–1139.

Dembroski, T. M., MacDougall, J. M., Williams, R. B., Jr., Haney, T., & Blumental, J. A. (1985). Components of Type A, hostility and anger-in: Relationship to angiographic findings. *Psychosomatic Medicine, 47,* 219–233.

deMendonca, M., Elliott, L., Goldstein, M., McNeill, J., Rodriguez, R., & Zelkind, I. (1984). An MMPI-based behavior descriptor/personality trait list. *Journal of Personality Assessment, 48,* 483–485.

Dubro, A. F., Wetzler, S., & Kahn, M. W. (1988). A comparison of three self-report questionnaires for the diagnosis of DSM-III personality disorders. *Journal of Personality Disorders, 2,* 256–266.

Duckworth, J. C., & Anderson, W. P. (1986). *MMPI interpretation manual for counselors and clinicians* (3rd ed.). Muncie, IN: Accelerated Development.

Duckworth, J. C., & Levitt, E. E. (1994). Minnesota Multiphasic Personality Inventory-2. In D. J. Keyser & R. C. Sweetland (Eds.), *Test critiques* (Vol. X, pp. 424–428). Austin, TX: Pro-Ed.

Edwards, A. L. (1959). *Edwards Personal Preference Schedule*. New York: The Psychological Corp.

Edwards, D. W., Morrison, T. L., & Weissman, H. N. (1993). The MMPI and MMPI-2 in an outpatient sample: Comparison of code types, validity scales, and clinical scales. *Journal of Personality Assessment, 61*, 1–18.

Eichman, W. J. (1961). Replicated factors on the MMPI with female NP patients. *Journal of Consulting Psychology, 25*, 55–60.

Eichman, W. J. (1962). Factored scales for the MMPI: A clinical and statistical manual. *Journal of Clinical Psychology, 18*, 363–395.

Endicott, N. A., Jortner, A. S., & Abramoff, E. (1969). Objective measures of suspiciousness. *Journal of Abnormal Psychology, 74*, 26–32.

Exner, J. E. (1991). *The Rorschach: A comprehensive system* (Vol. 2, 2nd ed.). New York: Wiley.

Exner, J. E. (1993). *The Rorschach: A comprehensive system* (Vol. 1, 3rd ed.). New York: Wiley.

Farberow, N. L., & Devries, A. G. (1967). An item differentiation analysis of suicidal neuropsychiatric hospital patients. *Psychological Reports, 20*, 607–617.

Faschingbauer, T. R. (1979). The future of the MMPI. In C. S. Newmark (Ed.), *MMPI clinical and research trends* (pp. 373–398). New York: Praeger.

Feldman, M. J. (1951). A prognosis scale for shock therapy. *Psychological Monographs, 65*, 10 (Whole No. 327).

Fisher, G. (1970). Discriminating violence emanating from overcontrolled versus undercontrolled aggressivity. *British Journal of Social & Clinical Psychology, 18*, 140–141.

Foerstner, S. B. (1986). *The factor structure and factor stability of selected Minnesota Multiphasic Personality Inventory (MMPI) subscales: Harris and Lingoes subscales, Wiggins content scales, Weiner subscales, and Serkownek subscales*. Unpublished doctoral dissertation, University of Akron, Akron, OH.

Fowler, R. D. (1979). The automated MMPI. In C. S. Newmark (Ed.), *MMPI clinical and research trends* (pp. 343–353). New York: Praeger.

Fredericksen, S. J. (1975). *A comparison of selected personality and history variables in highly violent, mildly violent and nonviolent female offenders*. Unpublished doctoral dissertation, University of Minnesota, Minneapolis, MN.

Gebhard, P. H., Gagnon, J. H., Pomeroy, W. B., & Christenson, C. V. (1965). *Sex offenders*. New York: Harper & Row.

Giedt, F. H., & Downing, L. (1961). An extroversion scale for the MMPI. *Journal of Clinical Psychology, 17*, 156–159.

Gilberstadt, H., & Duker, J. (1965). *A handbook for clinical and actuarial MMPI interpretation*. Philadelphia: Saunders.

Goldberg, L. R. (1965). Diagnosticians v. diagnostic signs: The diagnosis of psychosis vs. neurosis from the MMPI. *Psychological Monographs, 79*, 9 (Whole No. 602).

Goldfried, M. R., Stricker, G., & Weiner, I. B. (1971). *Rorschach handbook of clinical and research application*. Englewood Cliffs, NJ: Prentice-Hall.

Gottesman, I. I., Hanson, D. R., Kroeker, T. A., & Briggs, P. F. (1987). New MMPI normative data and power-transformed T-score tables for the Hathaway-Monachesi Minnesota cohort of 14,019 15-year-olds and 3,674 18-year-olds. In R. P. Archer (Ed.), *Using the MMPI with adolescents*. Hillsdale, NJ: Lawrence Erlbaum Associates.

Gough, H. G. (1948). A new dimension of status: I. Development of a personality scale. *American Sociological Review, 13*, 401–409.

Gough, H. G. (1950). The F minus K dissimulation index for the Minnesota Multiphasic Personality Inventory. *Journal of Consulting Psychology, 14*, 408–413.

Gough, H. G. (1951). Studies of social intolerance: II. A personality scale for anti-semitism. *Journal of Social Psychology, 33*, 247–255.

Gough, H. G. (1957). *California Psychological Inventory manual*. Palo Alto, CA: Consulting Psychologists Press.

Gough, H. G., McClosky, H., & Meehl, P. E. (1951). A personality scale for dominance. *Journal of Abnormal & Social Psychology, 46*, 360–366.

Gough, H. G., McClosky, H., & Meehl, P. E. (1952). A personality scale for social responsibility. *Journal of Abnormal & Social Psychology, 47*, 73–80.

Graham, J. R. (1977). *The MMPI: A practical guide.* New York: Oxford University Press.

Graham, J. R. (1978). Review of Minnesota Multiphasic Personality Inventory special scales. In P. McReynolds (Ed.), *Advances in psychological assessment* (Vol. IV, pp. 311–331). San Francisco: Jossey-Bass.

Graham, J. R. (1987). *The MMPI: A practical guide* (2nd ed.). New York: Oxford University Press.

Graham, J. R. (1990). *MMPI-2: Assessing personality and psychopathology.* New York: Oxford University Press.

Gravitz, M. A. (1970). Validity implications of normal adult MMPI "L" scale endorsement. *Journal of Clinical Psychology, 26*, 497–499.

Greenberg, J. S. (1985). Health and wellness: A conceptual differentiation. *Journal of School Health, 55*, 403–406.

Greene, R. L. (1978). An empirically derived MMPI Carelessness scale. *Journal of Clinical Psychology, 34*, 407–410.

Greene, R. L. (1979). Response consistency on the MMPI: The TR Index. *Journal of Personality Assessment, 43*, 69–71.

Greene, R. L. (1980). *The MMPI: An interpretive manual.* New York: Grune & Stratton.

Greene, R. L. (1991). *The MMPI-2/MMPI: An interpretive manual.* Needham Heights, MA: Allyn and Bacon.

Grosz, H. J., & Levitt, E. E. (1959). The effects of hypnotically induced anxiety on the Manifest Anxiety scale and the Barron Ego-Strength scale. *Journal of Abnormal & Social Psychology, 59*, 281–283.

Gynther, M. D. (1972). White norms and black MMPIs: A prescription for discrimination? *Psychological Bulletin, 78*, 386–402.

Gynther, M. D., Burkhart, B. R., & Hovanitz, C. (1979). Do face-valid items have more predictive validity than subtle items? The case of the MMPI Pd scale. *Journal of Consulting & Clinical Psychology, 47*, 295–300.

Hanley, C. (1957). Deriving a measure of test-taking defensiveness. *Journal of Consulting Psychology, 15*, 102–108.

Hansen, J-I. C., & Campbell, D. C. (1985). *The Strong manual.* Palo Alto, CA: Consulting Psychologists Press.

Hanvik, L. J. (1951). MMPI profiles in patients with low back pain. *Journal of Consulting Psychology, 22*, 350–353.

Harris, R. E., & Lingoes, J. C. (1955/rev. ed. 1968). *Subscales for the MMPI: An aid to profile interpretation* [mimeographed]. San Francisco, CA: Department of Psychiatry, University of California.

Hathaway, S. R., & McKinley, J. C. (1940). A Multiphasic Personality Schedule (Minnesota): I. Construction of the schedule. *Journal of Psychology, 10*, 249–254.

Hathaway, S. R. (1947). A coding system for MMPI profiles. *Journal of Consulting Psychology, 11*, 334–337.

Hathaway, S. R., & McKinley, J. C. (1951). *Minnesota Multiphasic Personality Inventory manual* (rev.). New York: The Psychological Corp.

Hathaway, S. R., & Briggs, P. F. (1957). Some normative data on new MMPI scales. *Journal of Clinical Psychology, 13*, 364–368.

Hathaway, S. R., & McKinley, J. C. (1983). *Minnesota Multiphasic Personality Inventory manual for administration and scoring.* Minneapolis, MN: University of Minnesota Press.

Haven, H. J. (1972). *Descriptive and developmental characteristics of chronically overcontrolled hostile prisoners.* Unpublished doctoral dissertation, Florida State University, Tallahassee, FL.

Hawkinson, J. R. (1961). A study of the construct validity of Barron's Ego-Strength scale with a state mental hospital population. *Dissertation Abstracts, 22,* 4031.

Haymond, P. J. (1981). *A new look at an old team: A correlational study of the Rorschach and MMPI with adolescent female delinquents.* Unpublished doctoral dissertation, Indiana University, Bloomington, IN.

Heist, P., & Yonge, G. (1968). *Manual for the Omnibus Personality Inventory.* New York: The Psychological Corp.

Herron, W. G., Guido, S. M., & Kantor, R. C. (1965). Relationships among ego strength measures. *Journal of Psychological Studies, 13,* 173–203.

Hoffman, H., Loper, R. G., & Kammeier, M. L. (1974). Identifying future alcoholics with MMPI alcohol scales. *Quarterly Journal of Studies on Alcohol, 35,* 490–498.

Hollandsworth, J. G. (1977). Differentiating assertion and aggression: Some behavioral guidelines. *Behavior Therapy, 8,* 347–352.

Hollandsworth, J. G., & Wall, K. E. (1977). Sex differences in assertive behavior: An empirical investigation. *Journal of Counseling Psychology, 24,* 217–222.

Huber, N., & Danahy, S. (1975). Use of the MMPI in predicting completion and evaluating changes in a long-term alcoholism treatment program. *Journal of Studies on Alcohol, 36,* 1230–1237.

Huff, F. W. (1965). Use of actuarial description of abnormal personality in a mental hospital. *Psychological Reports, 17,* 224.

Hutton, H. E., Miner, M. H., Blades, J. R., & Langfeldt, V. C. (1992). Ethnic differences on the MMPI Overcontrolled-Hostility Scale. *Journal of Personality Assessment, 58,* 260–268.

Jackson, D. N. (1975). The relative validity of scales prepared by naive item writers and those based on empirical methods of personality scale construction. *Educational & Psychological Measurement, 35,* 361–370.

Jarneke, R. W., & Chambers, E. D. (1977). MMPI content scales: Dimensional structure, construct validity, and interpretive norms in a psychiatric population. *Journal of Consulting & Clinical Psychology, 45,* 1126–1131.

Johnson, J. H., Null, C., Butcher, J. N., & Johnson, K. N. (1984). Replicated item level factor analysis of the full MMPI. *Journal of Personality & Social Psychology, 47,* 105–114.

Jurjevich, R. M. (1963). Relationships among the MMPI and HGI hostility scales. *Journal of General Psychology, 69,* 131–133.

Kammeier, M. L., Hoffman, H., & Loper, R. G. (1973). Personality characteristics of alcoholics as college freshmen and at time of treatment. *Quarterly Journal of Studies on Alcohol, 34,* 390–399.

King-Ellison Good, P. E. (1957). A psychological study of the effects of regressive electroshock treatment. *Dissertation Abstracts, 17,* 2064–2065.

Kleinmuntz, B. (1960). An extension of the construct validity of the ego-strength scale. *Journal of Consulting Psychology, 24,* 463–464.

Klerman, G. L. (1982). Practical issues in the treatment of depression and mania. In E. S. Paykel (Ed.), *Handbook of affective disorders.* New York: Churchill Livingstone.

Klopfer, B., & Spiegelman, M. (1956). Differential diagnosis. In B. Klopfer, M. D. Ainsworth, W. G. Klopfer, & R. R. Holt (Eds.), *Developments in the Rorschach technique: Fields of application* (Vol. 2., pp. 281–317). Yonkers-on-Hudson, NY: World Book Co.

Kobaṣa, S. C. (1979). Stressful life events, personality, and health: An inquiry into hardiness. *Journal of Personality & Social Psychology, 37,* 1–11.

Kobasa, S. C. (1982). The hardy personality: Toward a social psychology of stress and health. In G. S. Sanders & J. Suls (Eds.), *Social psychology of health and illness.* Hillsdale, NJ: Lawrence Erlbaum Associates.

Koss, M. P., Butcher, J. N., & Hoffman, N. G. (1976). The MMPI critical items: How well do they work? *Journal of Consulting & Clinical Psychology, 44,* 921–928.

Kranitz, L. (1972). Alcoholics, heroin addicts, and nonaddicts: Comparisons on the MacAndrew Alcoholism scale of the MMPI. *Quarterly Journal of Studies on Alcohol, 33,* 908–909.

Lachar, D., & Alexander, P. S. (1978). Veridicality of self-report: Replicated correlates of the Wiggins MMPI content scales. *Journal of Consulting & Clinical Psychology, 46,* 1349–1356.

Lachar, D., Berman, W., Grisell, J. L., & Schooff, K. (1976). The MacAndrew Alcoholism scale as a general measure of substance abuse. *Journal of Studies on Alcohol, 37,* 1609–1615.

Lachar, D., Lewis, R., & Kupke, T. (1979). MMPI in differentiation of temporal lobe and nontemporal lobe epilepsy: Investigation of three levels of test performance. *Journal of Consulting & Clinical Psychology, 47,* 186–188.

Lane, P. J., & Kling, J. S. (1979). Construct validity of the Overcontrolled Hostility scale of the MMPI. *Journal of Consulting & Clinical Psychology, 47,* 781–782.

Lebovits, B. Z., & Ostfeld, A. M. (1967). Personality, defensiveness and educational achievement. *Journal of Personality & Social Psychology, 6,* 381–390.

Lebovits, B. Z., Visotsky, H. M., & Ostfeld, A. M. (1960). LSD and JB 318: A comparison of two hallucinogens. *Archives of General Psychiatry, 2,* 390–407.

Lester, D., Perdue, W. C., & Brookhart, D. (1974). Murder and the control of aggression. *Psychological Reports, 34,* 706.

Levine, D., & Cohen, J. (1962). Symptoms and ego strength measures as predictors of the outcome of hospitalization in functional psychoses. *Journal of Consulting Psychology, 26,* 246–250.

Levitt, E. E. (1980a). *Primer on the Rorschach technique: A method of administration, scoring and interpretation.* Springfield, IL: Thomas.

Levitt, E. E. (1980b). *The psychology of anxiety* (2nd ed.). Hillsdale, NJ: Lawrence Erlbaum Associates.

Levitt, E. E. (1989). *The clinical application of MMPI special scales.* Hillsdale, NJ: Lawrence Erlbaum Associates.

Levitt, E. E. (1990). A structural analysis of the impact of MMPI-2 on MMPI-1. *Journal of Personality Assessment, 55,* 562–577.

Levitt, E. E., Browning, J. M., & Freeland, L. J. (1992). The effects of MMPI-2 on the scoring of special scales derived from MMPI-1. *Journal of Personality Assessment, 59,* 22–31.

Levitt, E. E., & Duckworth, J. C. (1984). Minnesota Multiphasic Personality Inventory. In D. J. Keyser & R. C. Sweetland (Eds.), *Test critiques* (Vol. 1, pp. 466–472). Kansas City, MO: Test Corporation of America.

Levitt, E. E., Lubin, B., & Brooks, J. M. (1983). *Depression: Concepts, controversies and some new facts* (2nd ed.). Hillsdale, NJ: Lawrence Erlbaum Associates.

Levitt, E. E., & Waddell, M. T. (in press). *The psychology of anxiety* (3rd ed.). Hillsdale, NJ: Lawrence Erlbaum Associates.

Lingoes, J. C. (1960). MMPI factors of the Harris and the Wiener subscales. *Journal of Consulting Psychology, 24,* 74–83.

Little, K. B., & Fisher, J. (1958). Two new experimental scales of the MMPI. *Journal of Consulting Psychology, 22,* 305–306.

Loper, R. G., Kammeier, M. L., & Hoffman, H. (1973). MMPI characteristics of college freshman males who later became alcoholics. *Journal of Abnormal Psychology, 32,* 159–162.

Lothstein, L. M., & Jones, P. (1978). Discriminating violent individuals by means of various psychological tests. *Journal of Personality Assessment, 42,* 237–243.

Lowry, R. J. (Ed.) (1973). *Dominance, self-esteem, self-actualization: The germinal papers of A. H. Maslow.* Monterey, CA: Brooks/Cole.

Lubin, B., Larsen, R. M., & Matarazzo, J. D. (1983). Psychological test usage in the United States: 1935–1982. *American Psychologist, 39,* 451–454.

MacAndrew, C. (1965). The differentiation of male alcoholic outpatients from nonalcoholic psychiatric outpatients by means of the MMPI. *Quarterly Journal of Studies on Alcohol, 26,* 238–246.

Mallory, C. H., & Walker, C. E. (1972). MMPI O-H scale responses of assaultive and nonassaultive prisoners and associated life history variables. *Educational & Psychological Measurement, 32,* 1125–1128.

Marks, P., & Seeman, W. (1963). *The actuarial description of abnormal personality*. Baltimore: Williams & Wilkins.

Maslow, A. H. (1968). *Toward a psychology of being* (2nd ed.). Princeton, NJ: Van Nostrand.

McClelland, W. A. (1951). A preliminary test of role-playing ability. *Journal of Consulting Psychology, 15*, 102–108.

McCreary, C. P. (1975). Personality differences among child molesters. *Journal of Personality Assessment, 39*, 591–593.

McGee, S. (1954). Measurement of hostility: A pilot study. *Journal of Clinical Psychology, 10*, 280–282.

Meehl, P. E., & Hathaway, S. R. (1946). The K factor as a suppressor variable in the Minnesota Multiphasic Personality Inventory. *Journal of Applied Psychology, 30*, 525–564.

Meehl, P. E., & Dahlstrom, W. G. (1960). Objective configural rules for discriminating psychotic from neurotic MMPI profiles. *Journal of Consulting Psychology, 24*, 375–387.

Megargee, E. I. (1966). Undercontrolled and overcontrolled personality types in extreme antisocial aggression. *Psychological Monographs, 80*, 3 (Whole No. 611).

Megargee, E. I. (1969). Conscientious objectors' scores on the MMPI O-H scale. *Proceedings of the 77th Annual Convention of the American Psychological Association, 4*, 507–508.

Megargee, E. I., Cook, P. E., & Mendelsohn, G. A. (1967). The development and validation of an MMPI scale of assaultiveness in overcontrolled individuals. *Journal of Abnormal Psychology, 72*, 519–528.

Megargee, E. I., & Mendelsohn, G. A. (1962). A cross-validation of twelve MMPI indexes of hostility and control. *Journal of Abnormal & Social Psychology, 65*, 431–438.

Meyer, G. J. (1993). The impact of response frequency on the Rorschach constellation indices and on their validity with diagnostic and MMPI-2 criteria. *Journal of Personality Assessment, 60*, 153–180.

Mezzich, J. E., Damarin, F. L., & Erickson, J. R. (1974). Comparative validity strategies and indices for differential diagnosis of depressive states from other psychiatric conditions using the MMPI. *Journal of Consulting & Clinical Psychology, 42*, 691–698.

Millon, T. (1981). *Disorders of personality: DSM-III, Axis II*. New York: Wiley.

Millon, T. (1983). *Millon Clinical Multiaxial Inventory manual* (3rd ed.). Minneapolis: National Computer Systems.

Millon, T. (1987). *Manual for the Millon Clinical Multiaxial Inventory-II, MCMI-II* (2nd ed.). Minneapolis: National Computer Systems.

Modlin, H. C. (1947). A study of the Minnesota Multiphasic Personality Inventory in clinical practice with notes on the Cornell Index. *American Journal of Psychiatry, 103*, 758–769.

Montgomery, G. T., Arnold, B. R., & Orozco, S. (1990). MMPI supplemental scale performance of Mexican Americans and level of acculturation. *Journal of Personality Assessment, 54*, 328–342.

Moos, R. H., & Solomon, G. F. (1964). Minnesota Multiphasic Personality Inventory response pattern in patients with rheumatoid arthritis. *Journal of Psychosomatic Research, 8*, 17–28.

Moreland, K. L., & Dahlstrom, W. G. (1983). Professional training with and use of the MMPI. *Professional Psychology, 14*, 218–223.

Morey, L. C., Blashfield, R. K., Webb, W. W., & Jewell, J. (1988). MMPI scales for DSM-III personality disorders: A preliminary validation study. *Journal of Clinical Psychology, 44*, 47–50.

Morey, L. C., & Smith, M. R. (1988). Personality disorders. In R. L. Greene (Ed.), *The MMPI: Its use in specific diagnostic groups* (pp. 110–158). Philadelphia: Grune & Stratton.

Morey, L. C., Waugh, M. H., & Blashfield, R. K. (1985). MMPI scales for DSM-III personality disorders: Their derivation and correlates. *Journal of Personality Assessment, 49*, 245–251.

Nash, M. R., Hulsey, T. L., Sexton, M. C., Harralson, T. L., & Lambert, W. (1993). Long-term sequelae of childhood sexual abuse: Perceived family environment, psychopathology, and dissociation. *Journal of Clinical and Consulting Psychology, 61*, 276–283.

Navran, L. (1954). A rationally derived MMPI scale to measure dependence. *Journal of Consulting Psychology, 18,* 192.

Nichols, D. S. (1984). *The clinical interpretation of the Wiggins MMPI content scales.* Unpublished manuscript.

Nichols, D. S. (1987). Interpreting the Wiggins MMPI content scales. In K. L. Moreland & J. N. Butcher (Eds.), *Clinical notes on the MMPI, No. 10.* Minneapolis: National Computer Systems.

Nichols, D. S., Greene, R. L., & Schmolck, P. (1989). Criteria for assessing inconsistent patterns of item endorsement on the MMPI: Rationale, development, and empirical traits. *Journal of Clinical Psychology, 45,* 239–250.

Norman, W. T. (1972). Psychometric considerations for a revision of the MMPI. In J. N. Butcher (Ed.), *Objective personality assessment.* New York: Academic Press.

Ohlson, E. L., & Wilson, M. (1974). Differentiating female homosexuals from female heterosexuals by use of the MMPI. *Journal of Sex Research, 20,* 308–315.

Palmer, W. G. (1970). *Actuarial interpretation of the MMPI: A replication and extension.* Unpublished doctoral dissertation, University of Alabama, Tuscaloosa, AL.

Pancoast, D. L., Archer, R. P., & Gordon, R. A. (1988). The MMPI and clinical diagnosis: A comparison of classification system outcomes with discharge diagnoses. *Journal of Personality Assessment, 52,* 81–90.

Panton, J. H. (1959). The response of prison inmates to MMPI subscales. *Journal of Social Therapy, 5,* 233–237.

Payne, F. D., & Wiggins, J. S. (1972). MMPI profile types and the self-report of psychiatric patients. *Journal of Abnormal Psychology, 29,* 1–8.

Pepper, L. J., & Strong, P. N. (1958). *Judgmental subscales for the Mf scale of the MMPI.* Unpublished manuscript.

Peterson, D. R. (1954). Predicting hospitalization of psychiatric outpatients. *Journal of Abnormal & Social Psychology, 49,* 260–265.

Pokorny, A. D. (1968). Myths about suicide. In H. L. P. Resnik (Ed.), *Suicidal behavior: Diagnosis and management.* Boston: Little, Brown.

Quay, H. (1955). The performance of hospitalized psychiatric patients on the Ego-Strength scale of the MMPI. *Journal of Clinical Psychology, 11,* 403–405.

Rawlings, M. L. (1973). Self-control and interpersonal violence: A study of Scottish adolescent male severe offenders. *Criminology, 11,* 23–48.

Reading, E. A. (1978). *The Rorschach and the MMPI: A construct validity study.* Unpublished master's thesis, University of South Florida, Tampa, FL.

Rhodes, R. J. (1969). The MacAndrew Alcoholism scale: A replication. *Journal of Clinical Psychology, 25,* 489–491.

Rich, C. C., & Davis, H. G. (1969). Concurrent validity of MMPI alcoholism scales. *Journal of Clinical Psychology, 25,* 425–426.

Rosen, A. (1962). Development of the MMPI scales based on a reference group of psychiatric patients. *Psychological Monographs, 76,* 8 (Whole No. 527).

Rosen, A. (1963). Diagnostic differentiation as a construct validity indicator for the MMPI Ego-Strength scale. *Journal of General Psychology, 69,* 293–297.

Rosenberg, N. (1972). MMPI alcoholism scales. *Journal of Clinical Psychology, 28,* 515–522.

Schill, T., & Wang, S. (1990). Correlates of the MMPI-2 Anger content scale. *Psychological Reports, 67,* 800–802.

Schuerger, J. M., Foerstner, S. B., Serkownek, K., & Ritz, G. (1987). History and validities of the Serkownek subscales for MMPI Scales 5 and 0. *Psychological Reports, 61,* 227–235.

Shaw, M. C., & Grubb, J. (1958). Hostility and able high school underachievers. *Journal of Counseling Psychology, 5,* 263–266.

Shekelle, R. B., Gale, M., Ostfeld, A. M., & Paul, O. (1983). Hostility, risk of coronary heart disease, and mortality. *Psychosomatic Medicine, 45,* 109–114.

Shipman, W. G. (1965). The validity of MMPI hostility scales. *Journal of Clinical Psychology, 21,* 186–190.

Sines, L. K., & Silver, R. J. (1963). An index of psychopathology (IP) derived from clinicians' judgments of MMPI profiles. *Journal of Clinical Psychology, 19,* 324–326.

Sinnett, E. R. (1962). The relationship between the Ego-Strength scale and rated in-hospital improvement. *Journal of Clinical Psychology, 14,* 46–47.

Smith, T. W., & Frohm, K. D. (1985). What's so unhealthy about hostility? Construct validity and psychosocial correlates of the Cook and Medley Ho scale. *Health Psychology, 4,* 503–520.

Smith, W. H., & Coyle, F. A., Jr. (1969). MMPI and Rorschach form level scores in a student population. *Journal of Psychology, 73,* 3–7.

Snow, D. L., & Held, M. L. (1973). Relation between locus of control and the MMPI with obese female adolescents. *Journal of Clinical Psychology, 29,* 24–25.

Spielberger, C. D., Gorsuch, R. I., Lushene, R., Vagg, P. R., & Jacobs, G. A. (1983). *Manual for the State-Trait Anxiety Inventory,* Form Y. Palo Alto, CA: Consulting Psychologists Press.

Spielberger, C. D., Jacobs, G. A., Russell, S., & Crane, R. S. (1983). Assessment of anger: The State-Trait Anger Scale. In J. N. Butcher & C. D. Spielberger (Eds.), *Advances in personality assessment* (Vol. 2, pp. 159–187). Hillsdale, NJ: Lawrence Erlbaum Associates.

Stein, K. B. (1968). The TSC Scales: The outcome of a cluster analysis of the 550 MMPI items. In P. McReynolds (Ed.), *Advances in psychological assessment* (Vol. 1, pp. 80–104). Palo Alto, CA: Science & Behavior Books.

Sundberg, N. D. (1961). The practice of psychological testing in clinical services in the United States. *American Psychologist, 16,* 79–83.

Sutker, P. B., & Allain, A. N. (1979). MMPI studies of extreme criminal violence in incarcerated women and men. In C. S. Newmark (Ed.), *MMPI clinical and research trends* (pp. 167–197). New York: Praeger.

Svanum, S., Levitt, E. E., & McAdoo, W. G. (1982). Differentiating male and female alcoholics from psychiatric outpatients: The MacAndrew and Rosenberg alcoholism scales. *Journal of Personality Assessment, 46,* 81–84.

Taft, R. (1957). The validity of the Barron Ego-Strength scale and the Welsh Anxiety Index. *Journal of Consulting Psychology, 21,* 247–249.

Tamkin, A. S. (1957). An evaluation of the construct validity of Barron's Ego Strength scale. *Journal of Clinical Psychology, 13,* 156–158.

Tamkin, A. S., & Klett, C. J. (1957). Barron's Ego-Strength Scale: A replication of an evaluation of its construct validity. *Journal of Consulting Psychology, 21,* 412.

Taylor, J. A. (1953). A personality scale of manifest anxiety. *Journal of Abnormal & Social Psychology, 48,* 285–290.

Taylor, J. B., Ptacek, M., Carithers, M., Griffin, G., & Coyne, L. (1972). Rating scales as measures of clinical judgment: III. Judgments of the self on personality inventory scales and direct ratings. *Educational and Psychological Measurement, 32,* 543–557.

Tesseneer, R., & Tydlaska, M. (1956). A cross-validation of a work attitude scale from the MMPI. *Journal of Educational Psychology, 47,* 1–7.

Toobert, S., Bartelme, K. F., & Jones, E. S. (1959). Some factors related to pedophilia. *International Journal of Social Psychiatry, 4,* 272–279.

Tryon, R. C. (1966). Unrestricted cluster and factor analysis with application to the MMPI and Holzinger-Harman problems. *Multivariate Behavioral Research, 1,* 229–244.

Tydlaska, M., & Mengel, R. (1953). A scale for measuring work attitudes for the MMPI. *Journal of Applied Psychology, 37,* 474–477.

Uecker, A. E. (1970). Differentiating male alcoholics from other psychiatric inpatients: Invalidity of the MacAndrew scale. *Quarterly Journal of Studies on Alcohol, 31,* 379–383.

Ullmann, L. P. (1962). An empirically derived MMPI scale which measures facilitation-inhibition of recognition of threatening stimuli. *Journal of Clinical Psychology, 18,* 127–132.

Vanderbeck, D. J. (1973). A construct validity study of the O-H scale of the MMPI, using a social learning approach to the catharsis effect. *FCI Research Reports, 5,* 1–18.

Van Evra, J. P., & Rosenburg, B. G. (1963). Ego strength and ego disjunction in primary and secondary psychopaths. *Journal of Clinical Psychology, 19,* 61–63.

Vega, A. (1971). Cross-validation of four MMPI scales for alcoholism. *Quarterly Journal of Studies on Alcohol, 32,* 791–797.

Wade, T. C., & Baker, T. B. (1977). Opinions and use of psychological tests: A survey of clinical psychologists. *American Psychologist, 32,* 874–882.

Ward, L. C., & Ward, J. W. (1980). MMPI readability reconsidered. *Journal of Personality Assessment, 44,* 387–389.

Webb, J. T., Levitt, E. E., & Rojdev, R. (1993, March). *A comparison of the clinical use of MMPI-1 and MMPI-2.* Paper presented at the meeting of the Society for Personality Assessment, San Francisco, CA.

Welsh, G. S. (1952). An anxiety index and an internalization ratio for the MMPI. *Journal of Consulting Psychology, 16,* 65–72.

Welsh, G. S. (1956). Factor dimensions A and R. In G. S. Welsh & W. G. Dahlstrom (Eds.), *Basic readings on the MMPI in psychology and medicine* (pp. 264–281). Minneapolis, MN: University of Minnesota Press.

Welsh, G. S., & Dahlstrom, W. G. (1956). *Basic readings on the MMPI in psychology and medicine.* Minneapolis, MN: University of Minnesota Press.

Whisler, R. H., & Cantor, J. M. (1966). The MacAndrew Alcoholism scale: A cross-validation in a domiciliary setting. *Journal of Clinical Psychology, 22,* 311–312.

White, W. C. (1970). *Selective modeling in youth offenders with high and low O-H personality types.* Unpublished doctoral dissertation, Florida State University, Tallahassee, FL.

White, W. C. (1975). Validity of the Overcontrolled Hostility (O-H) scale: A brief report. *Journal of Personality Assessment, 39,* 587–590.

White, W. C., McAdoo, W. G., & Megargee, E. I. (1973). Personality factors associated with over- and undercontrolled offenders. *Journal of Personality Assessment, 37,* 473–478.

Whitworth, R. H., & McBlaine, D. D. (1993). Comparison of the MMPI and MMPI-2 administered to Anglo- and Hispanic-American university students. *Journal of Personality Assessment, 61,* 18–27.

Wiener, D. N. (1948). Subtle and obvious keys for the MMPI. *Journal of Consulting Psychology, 12,* 164–170.

Wiener, D. N. (1956). Subtle and obvious keys for the MMPI. In G. S. Welsh & W. G. Dahlstrom (Eds.), *Basic readings on the MMPI in psychology and medicine* (pp. 195–204). Minneapolis, MN: University of Minnesota Press.

Wiener, D. N., & Harmon, L. R. (1946). *Subtle and obvious keys for the MMPI: Their development.* Minneapolis, MN: VA Advisement Bulletin No. 16.

Wiggins, J. S. (1966). Substantive dimensions of self-report in the MMPI item pool. *Psychological Monographs, 80,* 22 (Whole No. 630).

Wiggins, J. S. (1990). (From the foreword) In J. N. Butcher, J. R. Graham, C. L. Williams, & Y. S. Ben-Porath, *Development and use of the MMPI-2 content scales.* Minneapolis: University of Minnesota Press.

Wiggins, J. S., Goldberg, L. R., & Applebaum, M. (1971). MMPI content scales: Interpretive norms and correlations with other scales. *Journal of Consulting & Clinical Psychology, 37,* 403–410.

Williams, H. L. (1952). The development of a caudality scale for the MMPI. *Journal of Clinical Psychology, 8,* 293–297.

Williams, R. B., Jr., Haney, T. L., Lee, K. L., Kong, Y., Blumenthal, J. A., & Whalen, R. E. (1980). Type A behavior, hostility and coronary atherosclerosis. *Psychosomatic Medicine, 42,* 539–549.

Winne, J. F. (1951). A scale of neuroticism: An adaptation of the Minnesota Multiphasic Personality Inventory. *Journal of Clinical Psychology, 7,* 117–122.

Winter, W. D., & Stortroen, M. (1963). A comparison of several MMPI indices to differentiate psychotics from normals. *Journal of Clinical Psychology, 19*, 220–223.

Winters, K. C., Weintraub, S., & Neale, J. M. (1981). Validity of MMPI codetypes in identifying DSM-III schizophrenics, unipolars, and bipolars. *Journal of Consulting & Clinical Psychology, 49*, 486–487.

Wolff, W. M. (1955). Certainty: Generality and relation to manifest anxiety. *Journal of Abnormal & Social Psychology, 50*, 59–64.

Woodward, W. A., Robinowitz, R., & Penk, W. E. (1980, March). *Predicting substance abusers' return to treatment from first admission personality scales.* Paper presented at the meeting of the Society for Personality Assessment, Tampa, FL.

Wrobel, T. A., & Lachar, D. L. (1982). Validity of the Wiener subtle and obvious scales for the MMPI: Another example of the importance of inventory-item content. *Journal of Consulting & Clinical Psychology, 50*, 469–470.

Zarella, K. L., Schuerger, J. M., & Ritz, G. H. (1990). Estimates of MCMI DSM-III Axis II constructs from MMPI scales and subscales. *Journal of Personality Assessment, 55*, 195–201.

Zuckerman, M. (1979). *Sensation seeking: Beyond the optimal level of arousal.* Hillsdale, NJ: Lawrence Erlbaum Associates.

AUTHOR INDEX

SUBJECT INDEX

A

A Factor Scale (A), 31, 52, 92, 159
Adjustment, measurement of
  psychological, 68–71
  social, 71–72
Alcoholism Scale, see MacAndrew
  Alcoholism Scale
Alienation
  measurement of, 58–59, 139–140
  prognosis with, 66
Alienation Scale (4SOA) (Pd4), 21, 22, 28
Altruism Scale, see Conventionality Scale
Amorality Scale (9AMO) (Ma1), 22, 28, 30,
  58, 59, 62, 73, 78, 79, 82, 86, 93, 94,
  96, 114, 116, 120, 121, 123, 125, 146,
  147, 148, 151, 154, 158
Anger, measurement of, 59, 135–136
Antisocial personality disorder, measurement
  of, 78, 85–87, 89, 147–148
Antisocial tendency, measurement of, 58
Anxiety, measurement of, 52, 129–130
  social anxiety, 137–139, 155
Assertiveness Scale (Astvn), 45–46, 75–76,
  81, 86, 96, 98, 114, 116, 120, 125,
  145, 150
Atypical or mixed personality disorder, 90,
  153–154

Authority conflict
  measurement of, 59, 140
  personality pattern, 73–74
Authority Conflict Scale (4AC) (Pd2), 22, 23,
  25, 26, 28, 30, 58, 73, 75, 78, 81, 86,
  104, 113, 116, 119, 121, 122, 124,
  140, 147, 148, 150, 151, 153, 156
Authority Conflict Scale (AUT), 33, 45, 46,
  58, 59, 73, 74, 75, 78, 80, 81, 83, 86,
  94, 100, 109, 111, 116, 120, 122, 123,
  125, 140, 147, 148, 150, 151, 156, 158
Autism Scale (TSC/A), 37, 104, 105, 125
Avoidant personality disorder, measurement
  of, 83, 85–87, 88–90, 152
Avoidant tendency, prognosis with, 66

B

Bizarre Sensory Experiences Scale (8BSE)
  (Sc3), 22, 27, 28, 57, 84, 94, 95, 114,
  116, 119, 121, 123, 125, 131, 132,
  133, 152, 158
Body Symptoms Scale (TSC/B), 27, 37, 38,
  82, 85, 95, 104, 112, 116, 120, 121,
  123, 125, 136, 137, 151
Borderline personality disorder, measurement
  of, 80–81, 85–87, 89, 128, 149–150

179